Dutton

URBAN HEALTH IN AMERICA

URBAN HEALTH IN AMERICA

Amasa B. Ford, M.D.

New York
OXFORD UNIVERSITY PRESS
London 1976 Toronto

Library of Congress Catalogue Card Number: 75-32359
Printed in the United States of America

CONTENTS

PREFACE

American life is urbanized to a degree that population figures do not reveal, but the figures alone are telling. By 1970, more than one-half the population lived in communities of at least 15,000 and more than one-quarter in cities of 100,000 or more, while the proportion living outside towns and cities had dropped from two-thirds to less than one-quarter over the past 100 years. In our eastern and Great Lakes states, more of the population is crowded into cities of over a million inhabitants than in a comparable area of Western Europe. First migration westward, then northward and rural-to-urban, and now suburban expansion and the confluence of adjacent population centers have created a new kind of city, the megalopolis.

The main purpose of this book is to describe and evaluate the effect of this urbanization on the health of the people living in cities in the United States. Health consequences of the physical and social environment of the city will be assessed in the first four chapters, in the light of recent and objective information.

The convergence of people and resources in the city has also given rise to a complicated system of health providers and services, characterized by both unprecedented capability and unnecessary social injustice. How it operates, and to whose benefit, are questions that will be addressed in the next four chapters.

As in other countries, our state of health and our health care system have developed in ways that reflect the particular political and social character of the nation. Especially American is a strong commitment to individualism and free enterprise, which has expressed itself in the way doctors have clung to solo, fee-for-service practice, in our tendency to devalue individuals who fall by the way, whether because of laziness, lack of opportunity, or illness, and, on the other side of the ledger, in the way independent scientific investigation and medical technology have flourished.

A second social value that has had surges of strong support in the United States since the Declaration of Independence is egalitarianism and social justice. A widespread movement toward hygiene and sanitary reform before and after the Civil War established the principles of public health and gave substance to the claim that every citizen has a right to safe food and water and to the benefits of communal management of such health hazards as sewage and muddy streets. The distress of the Great Depression resulted in Social Security and gave new vigor to the drive for national health insurance and a national health system. The health program, however, was deterred by the opposition of the organized medical profession and only partially effected, under the impetus of movements for social justice in the 1960's, with the passage of Medicare.

A third democratic value, less prominent in American history than personal liberty and social equality, may yet furnish the essential basis for a health care system designed on a human scale and able to withstand the dehumanizing forces of the city. The traditional political term, "fraternity," may be redefined as the mutually supportive interaction of a small group of individuals, based on affection and shared values and goals, and harmoniously related to the larger society. Not yet agreed upon as a general principle, the idea is nevertheless gaining currency as we move toward more group practice, more team care, and, especially, toward a redefined family practice, which acknowledges the persistent importance of the family as a social unit and aims to reinforce its strengths by interaction with small groups of health care workers.

The complex problems of urban health defy simply solutions, but the city teems with possibilities. In the course of this analysis, many ideas, plans, and experiments will be noted. A scientific and rational approach, for example, suggests technological and managerial answers. The perspective of social reform, on the other hand, favors such measures as programmatic legislation, community organization, and consumer control. The conclusion that flows from a new emphasis on human brotherhood is that we must strive to understand and utilize the groups in which people live and work.

As a first step toward establishing general priorities and allocating our resources wisely, the following objectives will be defined and elaborated as an agenda for better urban health:

- a physical environment that will protect and support human life (Chapter 1).
- freedom from serious infectious disease (Chapter 2)
- a social environment that favors the development of human potential (Chapter 3)
- a decent life for individuals who are unable to support themselves because of age, disability, or illness (Chapter 4)
- equal access to good health services for all, not determined by ability to pay (Chapter 5)
- effective personal health care, provided by competent and interested persons (Chapter 6)

Finally, the analysis of the health care system in the last three chapters leads to the statement of another objective:

- human relationships within small groups of health workers and recipients characterized by affection and shared values and goals (Chapter 9)

The tasks required to accomplish these objectives are many and difficult, but unavoidable. Having cast our lot with the city, we must grapple with its harsh physical and social realities in order to build a more human habitation.

School of Medicine
Case Western Reserve University
Cleveland, Ohio

A.B.F.

November 1975

ACKNOWLEDGMENTS

The ideas in this book come from many sources, though I must take responsibility for their expression. I am particularly grateful for the intellectual challenge provided by Case Western Reserve medical students and for the keen skepticism and warm interest of Dean Frederick C. Robbins. The plan of the book originated during a stimulating sabbatical year with Professor J. N. Morris at the London School of Hygiene and Tropical Medicine. Professor Kerr L. White of The Johns Hopkins School of Hygiene and Public Health gave me indispensable encouragement and criticism during the writing. The National Center for Health Statistics has furnished previously unpublished mortality data. The labor of preparing the manuscript has been cheerfully shared by many, notably Carla Hochschild, John Henry Pfifferling, Elaine Allen, Marcia Manwaring, Hadas Greene, Eunice Horton, Mary Lou Sangdahl, Rita Kingsbury, Jo Merrill, Paul Alexander and the staff of the Cleveland Health Science Library. To these, and to many other colleagues and friends, and particularly to my dear wife, Daisy, I give thanks for encouragement, patience, and all kinds of help.

Amasa B. Ford, M.D.

1 AIRS, WATERS, AND PLACES

On approaching a new city, the physician in fifth century Greece was instructed by the Hippocratic writings to observe the physical characteristics of the place and its relation to the natural environment and climate, since different diseases are associated with different airs, waters, and places, and successful treatment depends upon observing and understanding these relationships.[1]

This is still sound advice. Many illnesses have uneven geographic distributions. Some illnesses that are concentrated in cities can be clearly explained as consequences of the physical environment that we have carelessly thrown up about ourselves in our haste to get on with industrial progress. For others, including some of the leading causes of death today, there is mounting evidence that the urban environment contributes either to the origin or to the severity of the disease. In this chapter we will examine how certain diseases are related to the airs, waters, and places of our residence.

LEAD POISONING IN CHILDHOOD

The story of lead poisoning in childhood epitomizes our troubled relationship with an artificial environment. In it we see how technology has accidentally produced human casualties and, at the same time, how a scientific approach and new technology can help prevent these deaths. At the social and political level, this story demonstrates that preoccupation with individual cases can blind us to a general health problem, while control measures illustrate the possibility of social action for better public health.

Lead was one of the first metals to be used by man. Its wide distribution and its affinity for sulfur make it readily available, mainly in the form of galena (lead sulfide), which can be smelted at low temperatures to produce the metal. Its malleability and durability recommended it for many uses. Ironically, its affinity for sulfur also makes it toxic to man, since it inactivates the sulfhydryl (SH) groups of enzymes necessary for the synthesis of heme, the oxygen-carrying pigment, and may interfere with other metabolic systems of cells. We have periodically recognized and then forgotten about the toxicity of lead since it was first described by the Greek poet-physician Nicander in the second century B.C. Lead has been repeatedly introduced into cider and alcoholic drinks by processing, storage, or consumption in soldered or lead vessels or pottery painted with lead-containing glazes. More recently, industrial exposures have resulted from the manufacture of batteries and tetraethyl lead, which in turn has led to reasonably effective protection for workers, though not for the public.[2, 3]

White lead ($Pb(OH)_2 \cdot 2\ PbCO_2$) is one of the oldest pigments known. For centuries it was manufactured essentially as in Roman times. A fast process for making it was introduced by Edwin Euston of Philadelphia in the late nineteenth century, and the United States became a leading producer of white lead. White lead was widely used to paint the homes and public buildings of the United States, where wood was the most widely available building material. Peeling lead paint forms chips, which taste sweet, and, today, children who live in old and poorly maintained houses eat them. This behavior has been called pica and defined as an abnormal craving, but it is so widespread among children, especially when they are poorly nourished, that the chief cause of childhood lead poisoning must be located in the environment rather than the patient. The ingestion of lead paint chips can result in an intake of 100 times the safe daily load for an adult. In the 1890's, two physicians in Australia–another frontier country –first called attention to the fact that children could acquire lead poisoning in this way, and it was described in the United States in 1914.[4]

Over the subsequent 40 years, some 20 to 30 cases a year were reported in large cities, and the mortality rate was high. Although the sequence of events that produced the disease was well understood, few people recognized the real magnitude of the problem. The fact that the first law requiring a warning label on lead paint cans was not adopted in the United States until 1959[5] can be explained by the fact that lead poisoning in children seemed rare to physicians who recognized it only in the advanced cases admitted to hospitals.

A recent development in laboratory methods, namely the introduction of atomic absorption spectroscopy for the accurate measurement of blood lead levels, has made possible for the first time large surveys of children living in old houses in the slums of large cities, such as Chicago and New York.[6]

Increased attention is being directed to the question of lead absorption because the metal is present in the exhaust fumes of gasoline engines and forms part of the complex of urban air pollution. The average atmospheric concentration of lead in downtown areas of large cities is two or three times higher than in outlying parts of these cities.[7] Blood lead levels in children have been shown to increase with proximity to major urban highways or exposure to heavy traffic density.[8] Another possible source of lead exposure for urban children is the soil of yards and playgrounds to which stable lead compounds have been added in the form of peeling paint or residues of fuel. The average blood lead levels in urban children and adults are approximately twice as high as those of suburban and rural residents.[9, 10]

A child in a dilapidated central-city house, therefore, lives with a mildly elevated blood lead. If, in addition, lead paint chips fall into his crib or he encounters a mouth-high window sill, he is likely to get a large dose. This intake, if it is continued for three months or so, may begin to produce the symptoms of chronic lead poisoning: lassitude, cramps, vomiting, and eventually, stupor, seizures, and, possibly, death. The surveys in Chicago and New York have found that at least 5 percent of children aged 1 to 6 years have elevated blood lead levels (greater than 60 micrograms per 100 milliliters). Such children, according to a 1970 statement by the Surgeon General, "should be referred immediately for evaluation as possible cases of lead poisoning."[11] How many such children are there in the United States? Applying the prevalence rates reported for New York and Chicago to the central city population of children under 5 years who are below the poverty level, we estimate the number as 47,000. Using a different definition of "elevated blood level" (40 micrograms per 100 milliliters), Gilsinn, in 1972, estimated that there were 600,000 children under 6 years with such blood levels in 241 cities of the United States.[12]

A method of treating lead poisoning is available. It consists of mobilizing and removing lead from the body by means of chelating agents, which were first developed in World War II as a treatment for persons exposed to arsenic-containing, poisonous gases. The mortality of severe lead poisoning has been dramatically reduced, but at least one-quarter of the survivors have lasting brain damage,[13] and there is reason to suspect that lesser degrees of lead poisoning produce lesser degrees of metabolic disturbance and neurological damage.[14]

Thus, in the last few years, an extensive urban plague has been brought to public attention. The customary medical practice of waiting until a case "presents" has largely hidden the problem of lead poisoning from us, and the act of returning a child to an unmodified environment stands condemned as gross negligence. How can we protect a child from his own home? Fortunately, a quirk of industrial evolution has set some limits to the danger. Beginning about 1940, paint manufacturers began to replace white lead in paints with titanium dioxide not because it was less toxic but because it had superior covering and coloring qualities and was cheaper. Today, lead is rarely used in paints for interior decorating, and the danger from that source presumably will endure only as long as the old lead paint surfaces last. Meanwhile, lead poisoning continues to occur.

If we accept better health for all as a national goal, it is plain that one item on the agenda must be to protect children from involuntary intoxication by lead paint, which still appears to be the major source of lead. This is a sizable task, but one we know how to perform. A complete program of prevention calls for action by physicians, public health officials, local government, and, probably, also national government. Two kinds of action are needed: scientific and social. First, we need cheaper and more accurate methods for surveillance. The usual method of measuring blood levels requires the drawing of 10 milliliters of blood from the vein of every potentially exposed child, but a micro method that uses a drop of finger blood is being developed, and it makes regular surveys more feasible. Next, all physicians who care for children must be alerted to the danger of lead poisoning and must understand their responsibility in detection of the disease and prevention of its development. They must also think and act as public health agents. The physician can sometimes prevent the child's returning to a toxic environment by persuading the parents to remove or cover lead paint, or to move to a safer home, and by reporting the case to public health officials. Every city—and probably some rural areas, such as those in which migrant worker camps are located[15]—should make the disease reportable and provide personnel and money, as New York did for a few years, for inspection and renovation of old housing. The fact that existing housing codes are poorly enforced emphasizes the need for those in possession of the information to transmit it to the public, even though this may involve scientists in the unaccustomed roles of health advocate. Finally, national legislation for the support of case-finding surveys and environmental rehabilitation has been only partially funded. Warning labels on lead paint containers are also required by a recent federal law, but the task of enforcement still lies ahead.

Toxicologists and physicians who have been aware of this problem for many years are not optimistic about the elimination of the lead paint hazard. The task of eliminating old lead paint from all urban houses seems impossibly laborious and costly, and recent studies implicate additional sources of exposure. Nonetheless, childhood lead poisoning is only one of several health hazards of the urban environment we are just beginning to confront, and some of the others are less well understood and potentially more dangerous.

MEASURING URBAN HEALTH

In order to think clearly about urban health, we need to define two complex ideas: "city" and "health." In the interests of continuity, the detailed discussion these terms require is placed in Appendix A, and the selected definitions will be summarized briefly here.

Health, at present, is measured indirectly by the absence or reduction of preventable deaths and illness and of disability. The concept of positive health, expressed in the charter of the World Health Organization, is a high ideal, and more will be said about it in later chapters. What we have at hand to work with, however, are mortality rates, based on death certificates and the decennial census, and rates of morbidity and use of services, obtained from national health examination and health interview surveys. These are the basic data, which can be supplemented by more detailed but less extensive measurements of death, disease, symptoms, and health-related behavior from special surveys and public health reports when they are available.

Cities

An operational definition of "city" that permits comparison of the health characteristics of the central city with those of suburban and rural areas is the Standard Metropolitan Statistical Area (SMSA). The SMSA is a county or group of contiguous counties containing at least one city of 50,000 inhabitants or more. Contiguous counties are included if, according to specified criteria, they are essentially metropolitan in character and are socially and economically integrated with the central city. Using this definition, we can examine the health characteristics of the United States population in three segments: central city counties, contiguous counties, which will be called suburban counties, and non-metropolitan counties.

The SMSA definition has some definite disadvantages, such as the facts that the "central city" county often includes the inner ring of suburbs and that "non-metropolitan" counties may include towns and small cities. But it is a workable definition, which is being used increasingly to classify health statistics. Since it includes population size, political structure, and social and economic relationships, it also permits some comparison of health factors with the important social and economic features of the urban environment (Appendix A).

Mortality

Mortality rates for specific diseases, subdivided by age, race, sex, and the three geographic segments, have been provided for this study by the National Center for Health Statistics (Appendix B). Uniform graphs based on these data give us a starting point for defining important health problems. Age-adjusted rates for deaths from all causes will be presented. Unless otherwise noted in the text, the geographic pattern shown in the figures is also demonstrable for age-adjusted rates in each sex and in the white and "all other" populations separately. The differences observed are highly significant statistically because of the large numbers of cases on which these national rates are based.

The data we will be considering are nevertheless limited, faulty, and often insufficient to bear the weight of important social decisions. They are not the best information we are capable of producing, and other countries, such as Sweden and the United Kingdom, produce better health statistics. It is striking that the businessman and the banker have access to a steady flow of economic figures—weekly and monthly rates of production, employment, and taxation, plus carefully computed trends and indices—while the publication of national vital statistics lags by three years, data from the National Health Survey are published sporadically and unpredictably, and there simply are no figures on suburban infant mortality to compare with the figures for inner city slums. It is sometimes difficult for someone who has not made the search to believe that we are so badly informed on matters that affect us so directly. Better statistics on health and social welfare are a prerequisite for better urban health, and this must be part of our technological agenda.[16] Meanwhile, let us look at the information we have.

Urban diseases

The average person living in a central city county of the United States faces a 9 percent greater chance of dying in a given year than his fellow citizens who live in adjacent suburban counties and a 1.5 percent higher chance than residents of non-metropolitan counties (Fig. 1.1). The figures shown are adjusted for differences in age distribution, and the same pattern can be observed in both sexes. During the decade 1960–1970, over-all age-adjusted mortality dropped 6.6 percent in central city counties, 6.3 percent in suburban counties, and only 2.8 percent in counties outside the SMSA, bringing the rates for central city and non-metropolitan counties so close that non-metropolitan rates are actually slightly higher when the races are considered separately. The differences demonstrated here represent many human lives. If the most favorable mortality rates in the nation, those of the suburbs, could have been matched in the country as a whole, 391,533 fewer persons would have died in the United States in 1970.

What do these differences mean? Are there specific urban diseases–or urban-related conditions–produced by the physical or social environment of the city? Does residence in the modern American city bring out latent illness or aggravate established disease? What part, if any, do health services play in producing this differential pattern, with the highest mortality rate in the central cities and the lowest in suburban counties?

In order to attempt answers to these complex questions we will have to take a more detailed look at some poorly understood disease processes and how they develop. Few urban-related diseases bear as clear a relationship to the environment as lead poisoning. But the effort to search out other disease-environment relationships is justified by the fact that today the leading causes of death, including some types of lung disease, cancer, and arteriosclerotic heart disease, show a distinct urban preponderance.

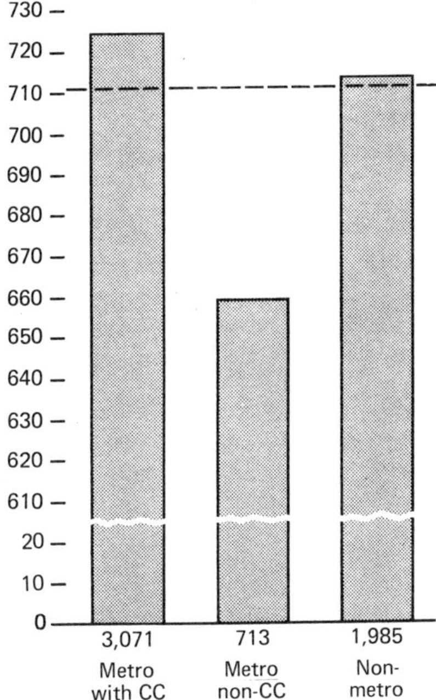

Fig. 1.1. **All causes of death:** age-adjusted annual mortality rates (U.S.,) 1969–1971, by county of residence. Ordinate, deaths per 100,000 population, (age-adjusted); dashed line, rate for the entire United States. Numbers below each bar are total number of deaths attributed to the cause specified in the United States for the three years. The last 3 digits are omitted in this figure and in Fig. 1.7 A and B. Causes of death in subsequent figures of the same form are classified according to International Classification of Diseases, Adapted (ICDA), 8th Revision, 1968. Counties are grouped as defined in text: metropolitan with central city (CC), metropolitan without central city, and non-metropolitan. (See Appendix A for definitions and Appendix B, Table 1, for data on deaths by residence, sex, and color.)

The relationship of respiratory diseases to the urban environment is of particular interest. Pneumonia and tuberculosis mortality rates are highest in the central city and lowest in the suburbs (Fig. 1.2). Death rates from all types of neoplasm of the respiratory tract, on the other hand, show a direct relationship to urbanization which, as we will see later, characterizes most cancers (Fig. 1.3).

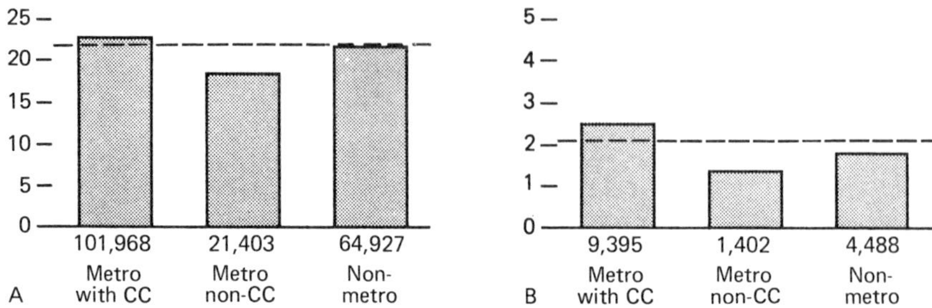

Fig. 1.2 **Deaths attributed to** (A) **influenza and pneumonia** (ICDA 470-474 and 480-486) **and** (B) **all forms of tuberculosis** (ICDA 010-019): age-adjusted annual mortality rates (U.S.), 1969–1971, by county of residence. (Cf. Fig. 1.1 and Appendix B, Tables 2 and 18.)

Chronic, non-malignant diseases of the respiratory tract present complicated diagnostic and semantic problems. The reported rates of death from chronic bronchitis and emphysema, which have in the past been low in the United States compared to Great Britain, have recently been rising more rapidly than the rates for any other disease. Some of the rise is apparent only, being attributable to more precise terminology and better diagnosis of a common condition that resembles and overlaps with other dis-

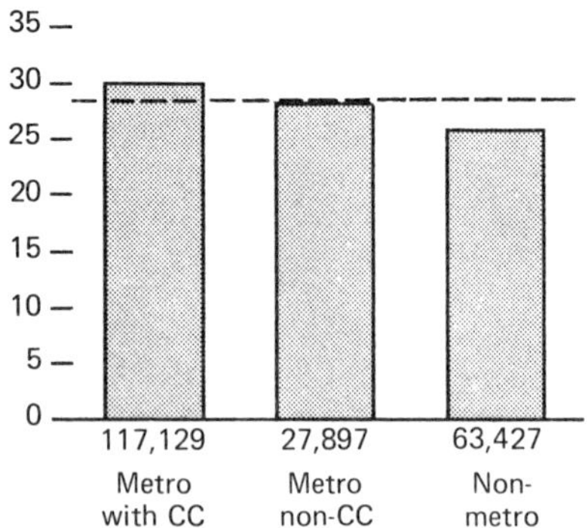

Fig. 1.3 **Deaths attributed to malignant neoplasm of respiratory system** (ICDA 160-163): age-adjusted annual mortality rates (U.S.), 1969–1971, by county of residence. (Cf. Fig. 1.1 and Appendix B, Table 6.)

eases.[17] Some of the increase may be related to increased cigarette smoking. Chronic bronchitis and emphysema showed the highest mortality rates in the central city and the lowest rates outside the metropolitan areas in 1960, but these conditions were not reported separately for 1970. The prevalence of chronic bronchitis among military inductees and parents of school children has been shown in several surveys to be higher in areas of greater and more frequent air pollution, and the effect of air pollution as a cause of chronic respiratory disease in large urban areas is estimated to be comparable to the effect of moderate smoking.[18]

Because of the obvious effects of inhaled smoke and irritant gases on the respiratory tract, efforts to relate human health to the urban environment have been concentrated on air pollution and its relationship to acute and chronic pulmonary disease. The subject has been extensively studied, particularly in Great Britain since the disastrous London smog of 1952, but also in such cities of the United States as Los Angeles, Buffalo, New York, and Chicago. Detailed, recent reviews are available,[19, 20, 21, 22] and our present understanding of the problem can be summarized briefly: "It seems probable that sufficient exposure to air pollution is a causal factor in chronic bronchitis and emphysema, but the likelihood must clearly be different in different locations."[19] The evidence for this relationship is more convincing for Great Britain than for the United States. Smokers and persons with preexisting heart and lung disease are particularly susceptible. The substances most frequently implicated, perhaps because they are most readily measured, are sulfur dioxide and particulate matter. The smog of Los Angeles has been particularly well studied. There, automobile exhausts, trapped in a geographic bowl in an area where frequent thermal inversions occur, react photochemically in the presence of sunlight to produce a peculiar type of noxious smog. The effects of air pollution on human health in Los Angeles and other similar cities include death from pulmonary disease, impaired breathing, aggravation of heart disease, sensory irritation —at times almost universal—the storage of potentially harmful pollutants in the body, and interference with general well-being. Goldsmith estimates that in California there are 100 to 500 deaths a year attributable to air pollution and that every citizen of the state is at least annoyed by air pollution sometime during the year.[23]

CITIES AND CANCER

There can be little doubt that urban air pollution damages the respiratory system. Evidence of a broader spectrum of dangers to health is also accumulating. Scanning the distribution of death rates for the most common diseases, one is struck by a remarkable pattern. Of all deaths in the United States, 61 percent fall into categories for which mortality rates are directly correlated with the degree of urbanization. That is to say, for every such cause, mortality rates are highest in counties with central cities, intermediate in suburban counties, and lowest in non-metropolitan counties. No diseases cause death exclusively in cities. A few, however, such as cirrhosis of the liver, exhibit mortality rates 100 percent higher in cities than in non-metropolitan areas, and many diseases show urban excesses of 10 to 20 percent.

Cancer mortality

The two leading causes of death in the United States, arteriosclerotic heart disease and cancer, show this pattern of progressively higher mortality closer to the central city. Within the general classification of cancer, all but two types (leukemia and malignant neoplasm of genital organs) have mortality rates that are correlated with urbanization. Cancers with this distribution account for 83 percent of all deaths from cancer, and 14 percent of all deaths. Rates for all cancers show the pattern strikingly, and it is seen in both sexes and in whites and non-whites (Fig. 1.4).

Cancer of the digestive tract also clearly exhibits a stepwise increase with proximity to the central city. The rates for cancer of the urinary tract and the breast, though similar for the central city and the suburbs, are distinctly higher than the rates for non-metropolitan counties (Fig. 1.5).

The respiratory, digestive, and urinary tracts are continually exposed to gases, liquids, and solids that derive from the imme-

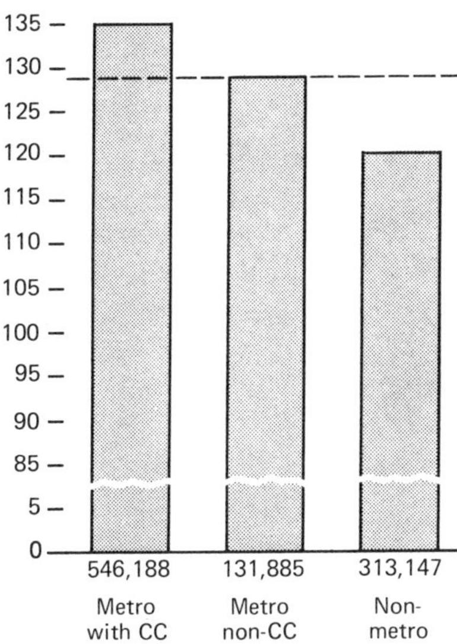

Fig. 1.4 **Deaths attributed to malignant neoplasms, including neoplasms of lymphatic and hematopoietic tissue** (ICDA 140-209): age-adjusted annual mortality rates (U.S.), 1969–1971, by county of residence. (Cf. Fig. 1.1 and Appendix B, Table 4.)

diate physical environment. The breast, at least in its secretory phase, is also in active contact with a number of substances ingested or inhaled from the environment.

In contrast, deaths from malignancies of organs and parts of the body not elements of a flow-through system show either no relationship to place of residence or a slightly lower rate in suburban counties (Fig. 1.6).

Is there a direct relationship between the incidence of cancer and the air, food, or water used by city dwellers? More careful scrutiny of the evidence is necessary before we can attempt to answer this question.

The fact that death rates from cancer are higher in urban than in rural populations has been confirmed in studies made in a number of industrialized countries during the past 20 years. In the United Kingdom,[24] Denmark,[25] Sweden, Japan, Czechoslo-

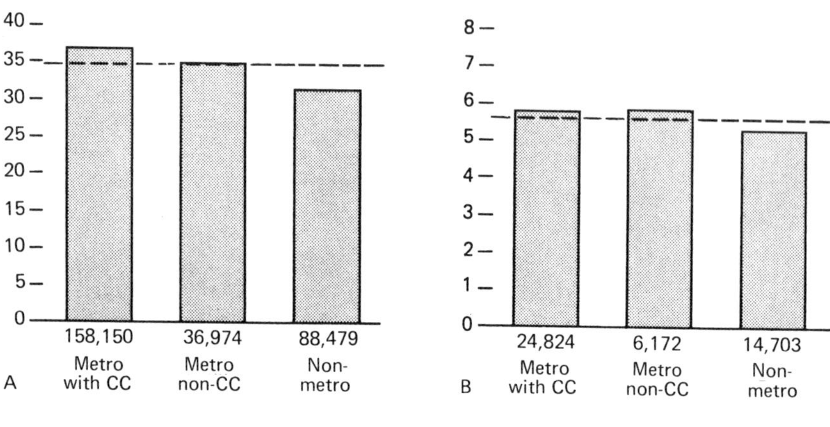

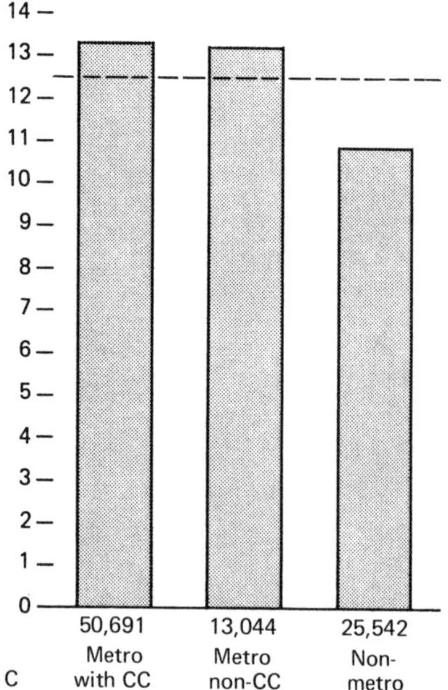

Fig. 1.5 **Deaths attributed to** (A) **malignant neoplasm of digestive organs and peritoneum** (ICDA 150-159), (B) **urinary organs** (ICDA 188, 189), **and** (C) **breast** (ICDA 174): age-adjusted annual mortality rates (U.S.), 1969–1971, by county of residence. (Cf. Fig. 1.1 and Appendix B, Tables 5, 9, and 7.)

vakia, and Italy,[26] for example, urban mortality rates, particularly rates for cancer of the lung, have been shown to be two to three times higher than the rates in rural areas.

In the United States, excess mortality from cancer has been demonstrated for urban, as compared with rural states.[27] Within individual states, including Connecticut,[28] Iowa,[29] and New York,[30] urban areas have proportionately more deaths from cancer of the lung, the intestinal tract, and other organs. Differences between urban and rural diagnostic skills and practice have been examined in these reports, but they are not great enough to explain the discrepancies.

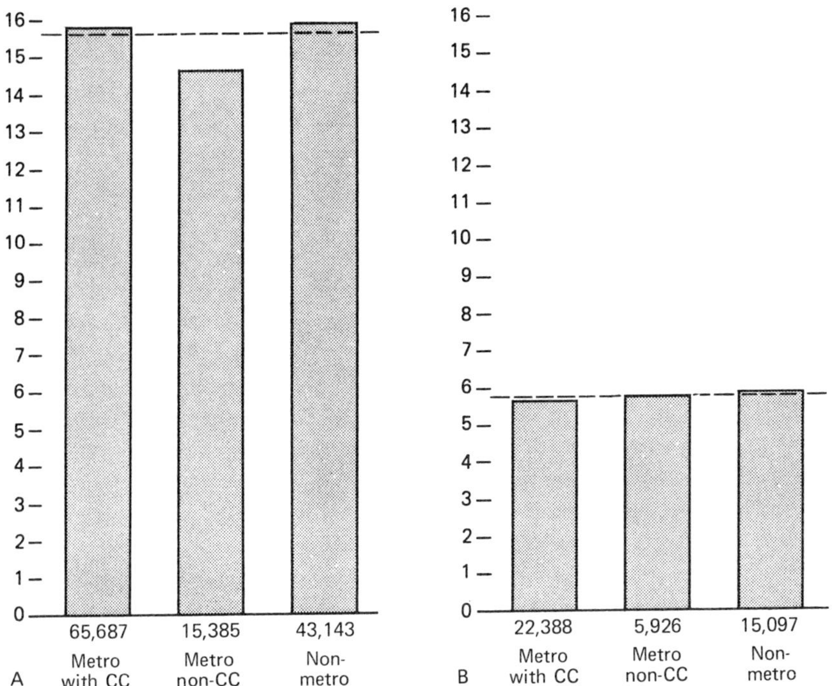

Fig. 1.6 **Deaths attributed to** (A) **malignant neoplasm of genital organs** (ICDA 180-187) **and** (B) **leukemia** (ICDA 204-207): age-adjusted annual mortality rates (U.S.), 1969–1971, by county of residence. (Cf. Fig. 1.1 and Appendix B, Tables 8 and 10.)

The distribution of cancer death rates within cities is also related to urbanization and industry. Mortality rates for all malignancies and for specific neoplasms, including those of the respiratory and digestive tracts, show a direct correlation with air pollution levels in Cuyahoga County (Cleveland), Ohio.[31] In Los Angeles, higher lung cancer mortality rates are seen among residents of certain heavily industrialized areas, where elevated levels of carcinogens have been demonstrated in the soil and air.[32]

Additional indirect evidence is the fact that for years after moving from the smoky air of British cities, migrants to South Africa appear to continue to show higher mortality rates from cancer of the lung than otherwise comparable persons born and raised in South Africa.[33]

In 1958, Hammond and Horn published the results of a prospective study of mortality among middle-aged American males that confirmed a higher rate of cancer of the lung among men of comparable smoking habits in the city as against the country.[34] The authors, however, stressed the strong association between smoking and cancer of the lung and confirmed previous observations by Doll and others.[24] Exploration of the smoking factor has dominated much research since. This line of investigation has culminated in the demonstration by Hammond and Auerbach that the smoking of non-filter cigarettes by dogs will produce invasive bronchioloalveolar tumors, including squamous cell carcinoma, one of the major types of lung cancer in man.[35, 36] With the evidence against smoking well founded, the graded relationship of cancer mortality to urbanization in cities of the United States now directs our attention back to the increasing concentration of carcinogenic compounds in city air and suggests that cigarette smoking is only one contributory factor, along with occupational and general environmental exposure, to urban cancer rates.

An urban factor in cancer mortality can therefore be distinguished, one not attributable to differences in smoking, in data from both Britain and the United States.[34, 37, 38] This distinction is important, since urban residents tend to be heavier smokers. In the United States, men who live in large cities experience a mortality from cancer of the lung two-thirds higher than that experienced by rural men and one-third higher than that observed in rural men of similar smoking habits.[34]

The urban factor in cancer

Only one of the current hypotheses about the cause of cancer, that of chemical carcinogenesis, offers a direct explanation of the increased rates observed in modern industrial cities. Heredity and virus infections would be unlikely to be directly correlated with urbanization. Furthermore, leukemia, which is the neoplasm that seems most likely to be caused by a virus, is one of the few malignancies that does not show a clear urban excess. Diet could be related to urbanization, but probably not in a symmetrical way consistent with the fact that suburban rates are intermediate between urban and non-metropolitan rates. Research on the molecular biology of cancer, though promising, at this stage tells us more about how malignant cells grow and differentiate than about the triggering stimuli that might be related to urban living. The inhalation of one or more specific cancer-producing substances offers the most logical link between these diseases and the urban environment.

Though the incidence of most cancers appears to increase with urban residence, there are enough differences in the distribution of tumors of specific organs and organ systems to suggest that such cancers are induced either by different carcinogens or by different kinds of exposure. The most and probably the best evidence has to do with cancer of the lung and bronchus. For this disease, the urban correlation, rising rates in industrialized countries, and information about the distribution and biological effects of known carcinogens are generally consistent with exposure to airborne substances by means of inhalation.[22] Cancer of the stomach also increases with increasing urbanization, but, in striking contrast with cancer of the lung, mortality from this tumor is rapidly decreasing in the United States and in other Western countries. No adequate explanation for this trend has been advanced. Efforts to identify a dietary factor have not been successful, though the interesting observation has been made that in some areas of high stomach cancer incidence, home-smoked or charcoal-broiled foods are frequently used.[39] Also, the consumption of cured fish in the United States, in contrast to most other foods, has been dropping steadily for at least 50 years.[40]

Inhaled particles, trapped in the bronchial mucus, are returned to the pharynx and then swallowed or expectorated as sputum. The intestinal tract, therefore, can be exposed to airborne substances. This mechanism may explain the urban excess in cancer of these organs, while exposure to foodborne carcinogens may be decreasing, leading to an over-all reduction in the incidence of cancer of the stomach in particular. Changes in the preservation and cooking of food may be of fundamental importance here. Since refrigeration and food processing are as much the results of technological development as is urban air pollution, it is again worth noting that the late fruits of the industrial revolution may be unintentionally helpful as well as harmful to human health.

It is not easy to relate substances suspended in urban air to a fatal human disease. The mixture of air pollutants is highly complex and varies not only in composition, but also with time, as traffic or industrial operations change the proportions of chemicals and as sunlight and temperature allow such components as oxygen and nitrogen to react chemically. Sulfur dioxide, nitrogen oxides, and particulate matter are present in large amounts in the air of every city. These substances are some of the commonest products of our accelerating production of energy by the burning of fossil fuels. They were among the first urban air pollutants to be measured regularly, and all three have been shown to have some epidemiological relationship to cancer mortality.

Sulfur oxides are produced by the combustion of coal, and, to a lesser extent, oil. Sulfur dioxide, especially when it is converted to sulfuric acid and adsorbed on carbon particles, irritates the mucous membranes and the ciliated epithelium of the respiratory tract.[41] Measurements of sulfur dioxide concentration in the air in Nashville and in 38 other metropolitan areas of the United States show some correlation with cancer mortality, but the association is, generally, not so strong as for other pollutants.[42, 43]

Oxides of nitrogen occur in large quantities in automobile exhausts and, in the presence of sunlight and ozone, form a photochemical smog, which can produce many mild, severe, and even fatal toxic effects, particularly in the lungs and bronchi.[44, 45] A consistent statistical association has been demonstrated between the concentration of nitrogen dioxide and deaths from several types of cancer.[42]

The concentration of particulate matter (dust or dispersion aerosols of particles) was one of the earliest measures of air pollution to be used. This type of atmospheric contaminant results from any kind of burning and is particularly characteristic of industrial smokes. Particles smaller than one micron in diameter are carried into the pulmonary alveoli, whereas larger particles are trapped in bronchial mucus and returned to the pharynx by ciliary action. The concentration of particulate matter in the air of American cities has been correlated with mortality from cancer of the stomach, prostate, and other organs.[31, 46, 47, 48] Since particulate matter is itself physically and chemically complex, and since it may function as a vehicle or associated irritant rather than as a primary carcinogen, more detailed scrutiny of the components of urban air will be necessary.

Carcinogenic materials have been identified in the atmosphere of virtually all large cities in which studies have been conducted. Some airborne substances that have been shown to be capable of producing cancer in man are those occurring in high concentrations in certain industries, in which the number of cases has called attention to the problem and led to intensive investigation. Asbestos, inorganic arsenicals, chromates, and nickel, for example, have been shown to be probable carcinogens for man[49, 50, 51] and are also regularly found in urban air.[52] Such materials may cause cancers in the immediate neighborhood of their industrial use, but their effect on the general urban population is unknown.

Incomplete combustion products of coal and oil include some of the most potent cancer-producing substances recognized. These are mainly aromatic hydrocarbons, though some aliphatic compounds share this attribute. For example, one of the earliest carcinogens to be studied is 3, 4 benzpyrene [benzo(α)pyrene, BaP]. This five-ring compound is a constituent of coal tar, occurs in tobacco smoke, and is found in the air of United States cities in concentrations of approximately 6 micrograms per 1,000 cubic meters.[52, 53] At least nine, large-molecule organic compounds found in urban air can produce malignant tumors in experimental animals.[52] Though they have not been proven to produce cancer in man, there is much evidence to suggest that they do. Stocks showed that the 3, 4 benzpyrene concentration in air roughly paralleled lung cancer death rates in communities near Liverpool.[54] Elevated lung cancer mortality rates are found in heavily industrialized areas of Los Angeles, where levels of benzo(α)pyrene in air and soil are also high.[32]

Recent experimental animal work has demonstrated that, though inhalation of organic carcinogens alone fails to produce malignancies, malignant tumors can be produced by adding irritant substances such as carbon particles, hematite, or sulfur dioxide.[44, 55] Such adjuvants may act by transporting the carcinogens in the body, inactivating normal excretion through ciliary paralysis, or increasing the susceptibility of the respiratory tissue in the course of cell loss and regeneration. Auerbach's successful production of malignancies in smoking dogs suggests that carcinogens carried into the respiratory tract by smoke exhibit a dose-response relationship and bring about a recognizable sequence of pathological change: hyperplasia, metaplasia, metaplasia with atypical change, carcinoma *in situ,* and invasive carcinoma.[35, 36]

Thus, the evidence strongly suggests, but does not definitely prove, that substances carried in urban air cause or trigger the development of several kinds of cancer. Before weighing this evidence, we must add to it additional information that points to a possible relationship between air pollution and heart disease.

CITIES AND HEART DISEASE

The stepwise pattern of urban increase in death rates is as striking for the leading cause of death, ischemic (arteriosclerotic or coronary) heart disease, as it is for cancer, the second most frequent cause of death (Fig. 1.7). Such a pattern is also seen with rheumatic heart disease. A major exception among diseases of the

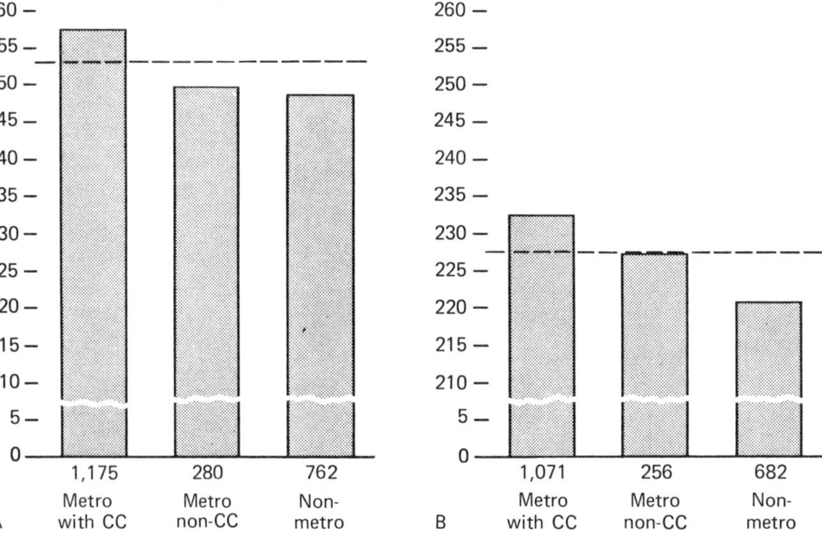

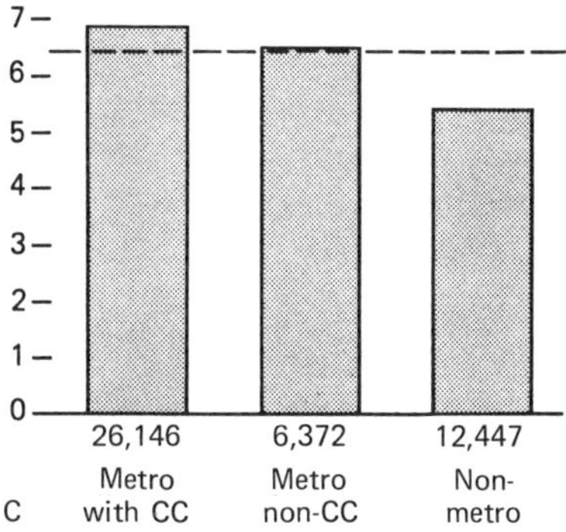

Fig. 1.7 **Deaths attributed to** (A) **diseases of heart** (ICDA 390-398, 402, 404, 410-429), (B) **ischemic heart disease** (ICDA 410-413), **and** (C) **active rheumatic fever and chronic rheumatic heart disease** (ICDA 390-398): age-adjusted annual mortality rates (U.S.), 1969–1971, by county of residence. (Last 3 digits omitted from numbers below bars in A and B. Cf. Fig. 1.1 and Appendix B, Tables 12, 15, and 13.)

heart is hypertensive heart disease, which is more likely to cause death in non-metropolitan areas.

Coronary heart disease is probably the main contributor to disease and disability, as well as the main cause of death, in the United States. Its prevalence, as measured in the National Health Examination Survey, has been found to be highest among men living in large cities and lowest among farmers.[56]

We have known for a long time that heart disease is associated with residence in cities, but this relationship has been overshadowed by the differences between high rates in wealthy countries and low rates in poor countries. Because the latter could apparently be explained by low consumption of fats and calories,[57] less attention has been paid to geographic differences in incidence within industrialized nations, differences that are probably not the result of a different diet.

Heart disease mortality

An opportunity to compare heart disease mortality rates in cities, suburbs, and non-metropolitan counties of the United States was provided by Manos and others who computed death rates based on the 1950 census.[58, 59, 60, 61] They found the same stepwise correlation with urbanization among white males and females aged 45 to 64 observed in more recent data. The greatest differences were in coronary heart disease, with less pronounced patterns among other types of heart disease. Geographically, the highest rates for both urban and non-metropolitan counties occurred on the eastern seaboard, along the Pacific Coast, and around the Great Lakes–that is, in the most urbanized sections of the country.[62, 63] Deaths among white men 45 to 64 years old were 20 percent higher in central city than in non-metropolitan counties. The observed differences could not be explained by differences in reporting, by errors on death certificates, by migration, or by institutional residence. Within New York State, over the same period of time, deaths from arteriosclerotic heart disease (but not from hypertension or stroke) showed a clustering of counties, with high rates around major industrial centers.[64]

In North Carolina, Tyroler and Cassel also demonstrated a striking urban gradient for death from coronary heart disease at two points in the 1950–1960 decade. Neither urban-rural differences in "diagnostic custom" nor selective migration of individuals with heart disease into cities could explain the findings.[65]

The incidence as well as the mortality rate of coronary heart disease in six counties of North Dakota was shown to be greater in white men of urban background than in men of rural background. Higher rates also occurred among geographically and occupationally mobile men, and all these differences were independent of diet, relative body weight, blood pressure, smoking, and parental longevity.[66]

A hint of how persistent the urban factor in coronary disease may be is provided by Sauer's demonstration that the cardiovascular mortality rates experienced by individuals who moved resembled the rates observed in the states in which they were born, rather than those of the states in which they died.[67]

The pattern of heart disease mortality may be very specifically correlated with the distribution of traffic and industry. Case fatality rates for patients admitted to Los Angeles hospitals with myocardial infarction are higher in areas of high air pollution.[68] Cardiovascular disease mortality was also related to air pollution, when age was taken into account, in an extensive study in Nashville.[69] In Cleveland, the highest rates of death from heart disease are shown to be concentrated in the very center of the city, with an intermediate zone extending south along the industrial valley. The distribution of both cardiovascular and cancer mortality rates is highly correlated with air pollution levels.[31]

The evidence strongly supports the hypothesis that there is an urban factor that increases mortality and probably morbidity from coronary heart disease. And yet it is remarkable that none of the major prospective epidemiological studies of this disease, such as those in Framingham, Massachusetts, in Tecumseh, Michigan, or a recently reported study in seven countries,[70] has examined this factor. The reason is probably one of perspective. Physicians searching for the cause of coronary disease first consulted their own experience. Clinical evidence, with some supporting epidemiological data, suggested disorders within the individual. Suspicion centered on fat metabolism, hypertension, and genetic and hormonal characteristics. Social and behavioral traits of individuals and groups, such as type of diet, lack of exercise, and smoking were studied next. These are the kinds of causes the practicing physician suspects from a careful observation of patients who have or who develop the disease. The study of these characteristics has established several important "risk factors" but so far has failed to reveal either an ultimate cause or an intermediate factor the control of which has clearly proven to be useful for prevention.[71] The search now widens. Extrinsic factors will probably be found only by examining the environment as well as the patient. Such studies, though not new, are increasingly important and have implicated a number of physical factors, including the mineral content of drinking water and pollutants in the air.

The urban factor in heart disease

Arteriosclerotic (coronary) heart disease is the type of heart disease that has been most clearly shown to be correlated with urban residence. The most common heart disease, it usually proves to be the main source of variation in epidemiological studies of all cardiovascular diseases. This discussion will therefore center on possible mechanisms that increase the risk of coronary heart disease for the city dweller.

Among the definite risk factors for coronary disease, none has been shown to be directly related to urbanization (i.e., highest in the central city, intermediate in the suburbs, and lowest away from the city). Hypertension, a leading risk factor, is actually more prevalent in non-metropolitan areas, and it causes a similar mortality in both sexes in all areas. Lack of exercise, diets high in saturated fat, obesity, and psychosocial "stress" are probably more typically seen in city people than farmers, but one might expect to find a wide range of these factors among residents of the suburbs as well as the inner city. The distribution of these factors by residence has not been studied–with rare exceptions[66]–and should be included in any future efforts to identify the urban factor(s).

Water hardness is an attribute of the external environment that has recently been shown to have a fairly consistent negative correlation with death from coronary disease.[72] Mineral content is a regional characteristic rather than one that varies with urbanization, however, and therefore it alone cannot be used to explain urban-related differences.

Air pollution is the most obvious suspect, and much available evidence supports this suspicion. Among the more readily measurable components of urban air, sulfur dioxide and sulfates show a positive correlation with mortality from arteriosclerotic heart disease that is independent of age, sex, and race.[42] Carbon monoxide, which has not been regularly measured in urban air pollution surveillance until very recently, has come under suspicion as a contributory cause of coronary heart disease.[73]

Case fatality rates from myocardial infarctions in patients admitted to Los Angeles hospitals were higher in areas of high air pollution but only during periods of relatively increased carbon monoxide concentration.[68, 74] In the study of air pollution and heart disease in Nashville, mortality from heart disease was related to air pollution among women and, when age-specific rates were compared, among men also. Carbon monoxide levels were not monitored.[75] A striking concentration of heart disease in a Japanese mountain village was found to be related to high concentrations of carbon monoxide in closed rooms heated by charcoal braziers.[76]

Cigarette smoking has recently been established as a risk factor for coronary disease.[77] City dwellers do smoke more, but urbanization and cigarette smoking are independently associated with coronary heart disease death rates.[78] Residents of large cities inhale carbon monoxide from cigarette smoke, automobile exhaust, industrial fumes and wastes, and fumes from home heating and cooking, and these exposures can be additive.[79]

The effects of acute and chronic carbon monoxide poisoning in man are under active investigation.[80, 81] The gas has a high affinity for hemoglobin. Both acutely and chronically, it can reduce the capacity of blood to deliver oxygen to metabolizing tissues. Regulatory adjustments to low oxygen levels in the blood are lacking when this condition is produced by carbon monoxide, with the result that body tissues do not receive enough oxygen.[82] When the blood contains 6 percent carboxyhemoglobin, the heart extracts less oxygen from coronary blood, and its anaerobic metabolism is correspondingly increased. Blood levels of carboxyhemoglobin this high and higher have been measured in smokers exposed to city traffic or to gasoline engines running in closed spaces.[83] A critical lack of oxygen may therefore develop in the heart muscle as a result of exposure to carbon monoxide during episodes of acute coronary insufficiency, and this series of events could contribute to the increased deaths among elderly people with heart disease that have been observed in episodes of sustained air pollution.

Chronic exposure to carbon monoxide may also contribute to coronary disease by other mechanisms. It has been known for 40 years that this gas can produce cardiovascular lesions in animals.[80] Recent work with cholesterol-fed rabbits shows that inhalation of concentrations of carbon monoxide comparable to those experienced by active and passive smokers and city automobile drivers will increase the deposition of fat on vessel walls, with the result that membrane permeability or enzyme activity may be altered.[84]

A sizable body of evidence, therefore, suggests that sources of environmental pollution, and particularly carbon monoxide-producing sources, are related to the development of coronary artery disease and to death from this disease. The main sources of pollution, of course, are the engines of our technology: the factories, automobiles, power and heating plants, which have been highly concentrated in cities of the United States and are now beginning to appear in the suburbs.

DOES THE URBAN ENVIRONMENT CAUSE DISEASE?

A search for specific agents in the urban environment that cause cancer or heart disease concentrates attention on external factors. We know from experience with infectious disease that finding such agents can lead to effective control. But the communicable disease model also suggests that the disease is more likely to develop if large numbers of potential hosts are in a susceptible state. Chronic diseases, such as cancer and heart disease, existed before there were any industrial cities, and people continue to die of them in rural areas and undeveloped countries today. Perhaps the agents, if there are specific ones that initiate these diseases, are no more prevalent than ever. Perhaps what has been altered by urban life is the host and his response.

There is some evidence that suggests a general urban factor, which increases man's susceptibility to several chronic diseases. Relationships between urbanization and mortality have been noted for nonmalignant as well as malignant disease of the respiratory and digestive systems and, in addition, for such dissimilar conditions as cirrhosis of the liver and tuberculosis. The concentration of chemicals in urban air can be used to predict the median age of urban populations in the United States as well as the mortality rates for cancer, heart disease, and congenital malformation. A positive correlation between air pollutants and median age was interpreted, in one such study, as the result of selective environmental pressures operating to eliminate susceptible individuals from the population at an earlier age.[42]

There are several biochemical and physiological mechanisms by which such an effect might be produced. For example, ozone and nitrogen dioxide react with animal tissues to increase cross-links in structural proteins and to increase cell turnover rates, both of which processes are associated with aging. Aging, and the diseases associated with it, may thus be accelerated by years of repeated exposure to oxidants.[85] Alternatively, individuals with an inborn relative deficiency of the enzymes needed to detoxify environmental substances may not survive the urban atmosphere.[86] Still other mechanisms by which environmental pollutants might increase susceptibility to disease are suggested by the fact that apparently inert vectors or irritants are needed in addition to carcinogens to produce pulmonary cancers by inhalation in experimental animals. One effect of many pollutants is to paralyze the action of the cilia lining the bronchi, so that particulate matter trapped on the mucus is not properly eliminated. By this mechanism and others, air pollution increases the susceptibility of animals to infection, which, in turn, may favor the development of chronic degenerative diseases.[87]

Living organisms have a great capacity to adapt to unpleasant or harmful environments by evolutionary change, and it is conceivable that over many generations modifications of the human organism may develop to make a significant number of individuals resistant to the urban environment. Some such adaptation may have occurred in the smoke-filled cities of nineteenth-century Europe.[82] Unfortunately, however, the slow process of genetic selection that has enabled man to respond to changes of climate and physical environment on a geologic time scale are outpaced by the explosive changes brought on by new technology within the memory of living man. We cannot rely on biological adaptation as an adequate defense against the toxic effects of many environmental elements in modern cities. Instead, we must deal directly with those elements of the urban environment most likely to cause disease. This we can already recognize as an enormously difficult and expensive task. As we begin it, we must be as certain as possible that we are getting at the real source of the trouble. Does the urban environment really cause cancer or heart disease?

In a wise essay on association, Bradford Hill observes that we never have conclusive proof that a factor in the environment "causes" disease. "All scientific work is incomplete–whether it be observational or experimental." Instead, we find different kinds of association increasing the likelihood that a relationship is real and that altering the environment will indeed alter the disease. Hill lists nine kinds of evidence that strengthen the possibility of significance in this sense.[88] Several of these criteria are already established for the connection between the urban environment on the one hand and cancer and heart disease on the other.

The *strength* of association is not so great as for more specific causative factors, but it is far from negligible. Urban residence, for example, is associated with an increase in lung cancer death rates of 33 percent, compared to an increase of 102 percent in death rates (all causes) in men who smoke a pack of cigarettes or more a day.[34] Such associations show great *consistency,* which is the second of Hill's criteria. The urban factor is recognizable in populations of comparable age, sex, and race. Associations have been reported from many industrialized countries and in studies that start with air pollution measurements as well as in those that set out to explain differences in mortality and morbidity due to heart disease and cancer.

Specificity is a weak point in the argument. Several different carcinogens occur in urban air, coronary disease is probably produced by different mechanisms than is cancer, and the incidence of both types of diseases may be increased in city dwellers by a change in their susceptibility rather than by specific agents. But Hill cautions against overemphasizing specificity. We recall that such a disease as syphilis produced confusing clinical pictures and gave rise to many remarkable hypotheses before the spirochete was discovered.

Temporality presents special difficulties in the study of chronic diseases. Lag periods between exposure to known carcinogens and the development of human cancers can be as long as 15 to 30 years. Current air pollution measurements, therefore, do not describe precisely the atmosphere in which the disease originally developed. The use of animal models permits some acceleration of exposure, but it also introduces other conceptual and practical problems. A parallel between industrialization, with its accelerated combustion of fossil fuels, and increasing mortality rates from cancer and heart disease is at least consistent with the hypothesis of causation.

A *biological gradient* is suggested by the stepwise progression of mortality rates as we approach the central city, as well as by differences between countries and states at different stages of urbanization. Gradients have been established in the production of animal tumors in studies of many constituents of urban air. Concentrated investigation of cigarette smoking in the last 15 years has demonstrated definite dose-response relationships between individual air pollution and cancer and heart disease. An increase of one microgram of benzo (α) pyrene per 1,000 cubic meters of air has been estimated to correspond to a 5 percent increase in the pulmonary cancer death rate.[89]

Hill also points out that biological *plausibility, coherence* with the known facts of the natural history and biology of the disease, and *analogy,* such as that between occupational exposure and exposure to the urban environment, all help strengthen the presumption of cause. On these counts, there is little reason to doubt that the physical environment of the city, if it is not the fundamental cause of these diseases, can at least prepare the biological ground for them or trigger their development.

Finally, *experiment,* though no more conclusive than any other evidence, can be convincing. Exposure of experimental animals to environmental substances has produced much valuable information and will undoubtedly contribute more. We can also take advantage of the "natural" experiments man is conducting on himself. Migration into cities continues to be a powerful social trend, bringing previously unexposed people into intimate contact with urban airs, waters, and places. New nations are directing their efforts toward increased industrial and urban growth, while New York and London have begun smoke abatement programs. Though we cannot say for sure that the air of our cities causes cancer or heart disease, we surely can no longer afford to disregard the mounting evidence that it does.

CLEAN CITIES

In public health, as in clinical medicine, circumstances may force action even when proof is incomplete or lacking. Today, the mounting circumstantial evidence against the urban atmosphere of American cities calls for immediate action. In the nineteenth century, we learned that it was possible to reduce the effect of infectious disease on the inhabitants of crowded cities by applying logical measures of hygiene, and that these measures could be applied even before the causative agents of such diseases had been identified. The relationship between gases and solids in the environment and human disease is now clear enough for us to set as a major objective for urban health: a physical environment that will protect and support human life.

Vigorous social and political action aimed at cleaning up the environment is already under way, and Ralph Nader has notified the National Air Pollution Control Administration that its efforts are insufficient. The Clean Air Act of 1963, with subsequent amendments, has resulted in the publication of detailed air quality control criteria for several components of the atmosphere, and the states have been required to formulate air quality standards and plans for implementing them. The beginning of a national air pollution surveillance system has been set up,[90] and it has been officially estimated that by 1977 we may expect to spend $12.3 billion a year and realize annual savings of $14.2 billion from the control of air pollution.[91]

Air pollution control is a good example of how the technological and scientific side of our culture contributes both to the problem and to its solution. Prompt action was possible in certain cities because technical methods of smoke abatement had been known, though not widely applied, for years,[92] and because low sulfur fuels could sometimes be substituted for high sulfur coal with relatively little increase in cost.[93]

National laws have reduced the competitive disadvantages for an industry that utilizes air pollution controls, and an important stimulus has been provided for engineering research in these areas. Now we need new, more efficient, and more economical means of reducing emissions and recycling combustion products. The nation is awakening to an "energy crisis." It is becoming apparent that attaching soot precipitators to industrial chimneys or exhaust converters to gasoline engines is not enough. We must think in terms of new kinds of fuel, new methods of producing energy, and, even, a system for rationing the use of energy and natural resources.[94] Enormous industries geared to petroleum production, the manufacture of automobiles, and the building of highways offer great resistance to such changes and tend to persist in wasteful practices, such as annual model changes and overpowered engines in the automobile industry.

The cost of unaccustomed environmental safeguards at first seems prohibitive, but present cost estimates may prove to be high in a field of rapidly developing technology. Changes to protect human health may also have economic advantages, as shown by the substitution of titanium dioxide for white lead as a paint pigment. In terms of air pollution control, economic benefits roughly equal to costs have been predicted as a result of the protection of property, "materials and vegetation," and health. A careful scrutiny of these estimates, however, shows that they are based on very little real information.

Among the many technical needs urban pollution presents is the invention of a new kind of balance sheet that will take into account the social cost of new and increased production in terms of human health and lives. According to one estimate, a 50 percent decrease in air pollution would reduce both mortality and morbidity by a minimum of 4.5 percent, with economic savings of $2 billion annually at present and $9 billion or more by 1977.[95, 96] But these too are shaky figures. The very momentum of the national surge toward air pollution control makes it urgent to press ahead with research so that we may know for sure which substances in the air are most harmful and so that we can compute benefits with a confidence based on more precise and convincing evidence than what we have reviewed in this chapter. We need, in addition to improved techniques of surveillance and pollution control, better, more detailed, and more current health information. No longer can we afford to wait while vital statistics drift from local to state to national levels, losing specificity as they go, entombed after four years in a thick volume, unrelated to the figures on environmental change and industrial production the costs of which they should spell out. We must invest in epidemiological studies of environmental causes of disease and death with the same sense of vital necessity with which we search for new sources of energy. Undefined sources of environmental danger lie ahead. Modern manufacturing and distribution are able to permeate our environments with new and untested chemicals in a very short time. Esptein has pointed to the critical need to screen new substances and to detect, investigate, and monitor widely distributed materials that are already known to cause cancer, fetal deformity, or genetic change.[97]

The tasks of detoxifying the world around us and of protecting ourselves from future inadvertent casualties call for vigorous action and may require investment on the scale now reserved for military defense. We can take courage for the effort from the fact that, as we shall see in the next chapter, past successes in the control of infectious disease have made the modern world safe and liveable to a degree that was unimaginable a century ago. The threats of lead poisoning, air pollution, and the many other dangers of the modern urban environment are surely as susceptible to rational analysis and planned control as typhoid, smallpox, and diphtheria have been.

2 PESTILENCE, PAST AND PRESENT

"Mankind have inhabited cities long enough to know from severe experience, that there are certain limits to the denseness of population which, when passed, lead always to disease and mortality." Dr. Gouverneur Emerson based this conclusion on mortality statistics for Philadelphia and Baltimore for the years 1821 through 1830. Almost one-quarter of the children who were born in cities in those years died before their first birthday, mainly from summer "cholera infantum" (infectious diarrhea), the "scourge of the cities," though comparatively rare in the countryside.[1] Today, only 2 percent of urban infants die before the age of one.

In 1844, Dr. Robley Dunglison, Professor of Medicine at Jefferson Medical College, attempted to explain high urban mortality rates as the result of "the confined and deteriorated atmosphere of the town acting in a manner directly unfavorable to human life; in other words, as a deleterious agent–a morbid poison."[2] Even as Dr. Dunglison wrote, a new instrument, the compound microscope with an achromatic objective, was beginning to bring into view a world of microbes, which previously had only been suspected. By 1876, Pasteur's long studies culminated in the demonstration of the bacterial agent of anthrax. The next year, he presented a full statement of the germ theory of disease to his still skeptical colleagues. Other discoveries followed with dramatic speed. In the next two decades, the bacterial agents of seventeen major diseases were identified; they included the agents leprosy, gonorrhea, typhoid, tuberculosis, diphtheria, tetanus, and plague, as well as the malaria plasmodium. The true nature of the "morbid poison" associated with crowded cities stood revealed.

A scientific chain reaction followed. Once an organism was identified, it could be spotted not only in diseased patients, but sometimes in fleas, mosquitoes, and other animal carriers as well. Then the leaders of the Sanitary Movement, who had been striving for 50 years to eliminate "filth" from the cities, knew exactly what they were after. The essential task defined itself. What was needed was a new kind of social engineering by new kinds of sanitarians, bacteriologists, epidemiologists, and health officers. It was an immense task, and at first it moved slowly. By 1901, life expectancy in New York City was still seven years less than the national average, and it was not until after the middle of the century that the difference became negligible.[3]

As nineteenth-century sanitation evolved into twentieth-century public health and preventive medicine, it altered Western society so greatly that it is difficult now to imagine what the urban world of the past was like. Figure 2.1 shows that, until a century ago, major cities of the United States lost about thirty of every thousand of their citizens by death each year. Though epidemics of cholera, smallpox, typhoid, and yellow fever produced spikes of annual mortality to 50 or even 100/1,000, the average rates changed very little until about 1890, when the application of new bacterial knowledge began in earnest. In the next 25 years, deaths in Boston, New York, New Orleans, and Philadelphia dropped from 25 to 15/1,000. Progress over the subsequent 50 years has been decidedly slower, with the crude mortality rate dropping only to about 9/1,000 today.

The major epidemic diseases have been eliminated from our cities and the chronic and complicating infections reduced to a shadow of the threat they posed a century ago. The change for

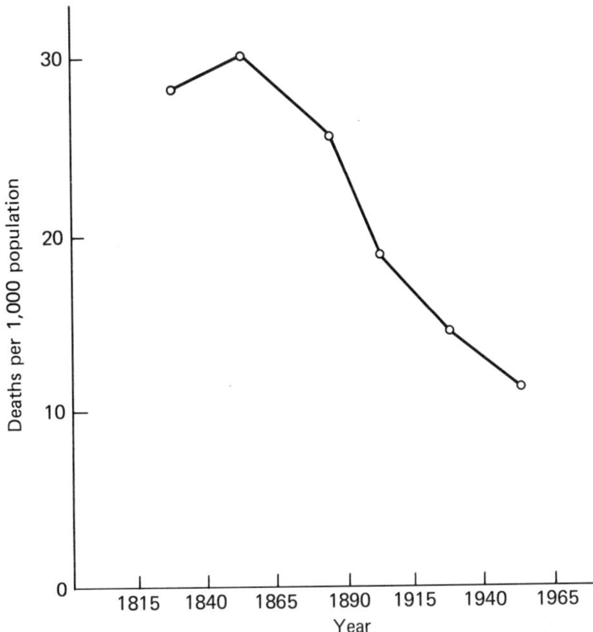

Fig. 2.1 **Twenty-five–year average mortality rates:** four large cities of the United States (Boston, New Orleans, New York, and Philadelphia), 1815–1965. Source: Hoffman in M. P. Ravenel, *A Half Century of Public Health,* APHA, 1921; Departments of Vital Statistics of the cities.

Philadelphia is shown in Fig. 2.2. If the mortality rates of the post-Civil War era still prevailed in that city, there would be 15,000 deaths a year from tuberculosis alone, and 28,000 from the other diseases. In fact, the number of deaths from these diseases that actually occur today is less than 2 percent of the projected adult figures.

The conquest of most communicable diseases in developed countries is a persuasive example of how scientific research and the rational explanation of observed biological and environmental facts can provide the understanding and tools necessary for effective social and political action. The development of the germ theory of disease was itself the outcome of a series of ideas, experi-

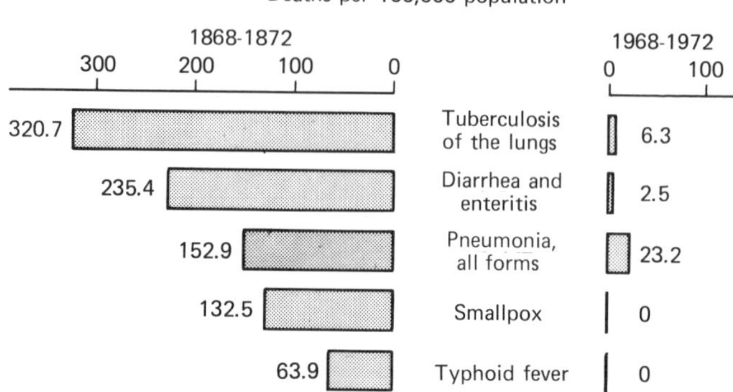

Fig. 2.2 **Mortality rates attributed to selected diseases:** Philadelphia, 1868–1872 and 1968–1972. Source: Hoffman in M. P. Ravenel, *A Half Century of Public Health,* APHA, 1921; Department of Vital Statistics, Philadelphia.

ments, challenges to established behavior and theory, and public quarrels in which "scientific" status and prestige often played as great a part as logical disputation. By patient and sometimes dramatized experimentation, Pasteur, Koch, and others finally convinced the doubters, and the way was open for the application of the new understanding.

The working out of the practical uses of new knowledge is usually assigned a less important status than basic scientific discovery. Granting that some experimental results are more charged with meaning than others, and that new insights, like the learning process itself, seem to advance by leaps rather than incrementally, it is still difficult to make a sharp distinction between what goes on in the mind of the basic scientist and in that of the innovative engineer or epidemiologist. The basic and the applied scientist think alike but work with different materials. Each must furnish himself with existing knowledge (Pasteur's *esprit préparé*), each must be alive to the clues around him, each must form hypotheses and decide which experiments to conduct; and those choices will be conditioned by the social and ethical bias of the experimenter. Finally, the experimenter must interpret his results in such a way as to be meaningful to others.

The work of the pioneers of American public health, almost inevitably starting with an urban problem, displays an objectivity and a willingness to experiment and be proven wrong, which must certainly qualify these workers as rational, if not always rigorously scientific. That these men and women were sometimes less than pure scientists can be accounted for by the strong political interests and the inertia with which they had to contend. Unfortunately, the mere demonstration of truth does not convince the world.

Two examples of the many skirmishes and battles that took place between the sanitarians and infectious disease will illustrate the interplay of scientific knowledge and social action. The first is the story of how Dr. Stephen Smith helped conquer both typhus and Tammany Hall and the second how San Francisco eradicated the plague.

STEPHEN SMITH: TYPHUS IN NEW YORK

When Stephen Smith, later to found the American Public Health Association, was a resident in medicine at Bellevue Hospital in 1853, a severe epidemic of typhus occurred. Ten of the staff of twelve residents suffered attacks, and two died. The survivors continued to struggle with the disease. Dr. Smith recalled:

> Upon examination of the records of admission of patients, I discovered that from one tenement house upwards of one hundred cases had been received. On visiting the house, I found a veritable "fever nest." The doors and windows were broken, the cellar was filled with sewage, every room was occupied by families of Irish immigrants who had but little furniture and slept on straw scattered on the floor. I learned that the house was the first resort of immigrants, as there was no one in charge and hence no expense.[5]

Though the germ theory was being discussed at the time, Pasteur's classic statement was not to be presented for another 25 years; the rickettsial organism that causes the disease and its transmission by louse and rat were not to be demonstrated for 50 years. Nevertheless, observing the fact that filth and disease occurred together, Dr. Smith hypothesized that elimination of the "fever nest" might eliminate the fever. This was a current idea, especially in England, though not a fully accepted one. In the same period, John Snow, in London, was tracing the connection between cholera and the distribution of contaminated river water, which he reported in his classic paper, "On the Mode of Communication of Cholera" (1849).[6] Like Snow, Smith acted on what he had observed. First, he went to the police, who said they had no authority to deal with such a problem. He next traced the owner of the tenement, "a wealthy gentleman living in Union Square," who flatly refused to improve the house. His next move was to present the problem to Mr. Peter Cooper, president of the Citizens' Association, which had been organized to defeat Tammany Hall. "Intense interest was manifested."

Fortunately, the Citizens' Association had already created a Council of Hygiene, to which Smith was promptly appointed. Previous efforts to pass health bills had been defeated because the unsanitary condition of the city and the incompetence of public officials had been denied, and proof was lacking. In 1864, Smith was commissioned to make a sanitary survey of the city of New York, which he did with such thoroughness that it was published in seventeen volumes—"the most complete work of the kind on record."

The facts he assembled were indisputable. There was no effective sanitary administration in the city. Posts were filled by politicians, who were totally lacking in medical or scientific training. What money was spent went in patronage to hire "health wardens," who were generally saloon-keepers. A Health Commission existed but had few defined duties. The picture of New York's poor, packed by the hundreds into neglected tenements, breathing the air from overflowing privies, making their way past piles of rotting garbage to airless and lightless basements was vividly recalled by Dr. Smith in 1911 in his memoir, *The City That Was.*[7]

With legal assistance, Smith drafted a Metropolitan Health Bill, modeled on the English Sanitary Laws, which was presented to the state legislature. In spite of all the evidence, the bill failed to pass. The committee now undertook a campaign of public education. With the campaign reinforced by the threat of an epidemic of cholera in Europe, the bill was quickly put through in 1866. A Metropolitan Health Board was immediately organized and was able to identify and quarantine the few cases of cholera that reached the city that year. Dr. Smith, writing in 1921, recalled

> The result of this new experience in the treatment of cholera was public confidence in the power of the Board to control and suppress the spread of contagious diseases. People who had fled from the city for safety returned: business was generally resumed, and for half a century cholera has excited little or no alarm here, even when it reaches Europe in its world-wide itinerary.[8]

Smith and other health reformers of the recent past performed great and successful scientific experiments. Starting with a hypothesis, crude at first, but progressively refined by new information, they made objective observations that led to specific experimental procedures: quarantine and general sanitation at first, later the eradication of specific vectors and mass immunization. The results of these changes were objectively evaluated by means of before and after figures and by comparing rates in protected cities with rates in those cities where public health measures had not been taken. It is an ironic development that the success of these experiments has been so complete that, since we no longer see epidemic disease in American cities, we are beginning to forget what they taught us.

But can we hope to conquer such contemporary urban plagues as air pollution without a powerful scientific weapon like the germ theory? The career of Stephen Smith shows us that major public health problems are clear enough in their general outline to permit effective action well before research has worked out the details of the mechanism. It is as evident today that the products of combustion are sickening and killing the residents of American cities as it was in 1853 that garbage, excrement, and other "filth" was sickening and killing the citizens of New York.

RUPERT BLUE: PLAGUE IN SAN FRANCISCO

The eradication of plague from San Francisco in 1909 is an example of how effective public health action can be when based on a thorough understanding of a specific disease.

An outbreak of bubonic plague claimed 121 lives in San Francisco in 1900. The plague bacillus had been identified in 1894, and its reservoir in rats and transmission to man by the rat flea was recognized soon thereafter. With this information, the first outbreak of the disease in San Francisco, which was confined to Chinatown, was controlled by 1904 by exterminating rats and by cleaning and repairing the buildings that had harbored them.

The earthquake and fire of 1906, though they seemed to have "sterilized" the city, in fact, broke sewer lines and created rubble where rats flourished. In May, 1907, with the cleanup and rebuilding in full swing, a sick man in a stupor was taken to the Marine Hospital from a tug in the bay. His disease was recognized as the plague, but he died without rousing enough to tell where he had been. The tug left port before the crew could be questioned, and soon thereafter it was lost off the Mendicino County Coast. The next case did not occur until August 12. Before the month was over, 14 people fell ill with the disease, and cases were scattered widely over the city. By September, 55 persons were infected, and the Mayor called on President Theodore Roosevelt for help. The Surgeon General ordered Passed Assistant Surgeon Rupert Blue of the United States Public Health and Marine Hospital Service to take charge of the situation.

The story of how Dr. Blue organized the entire city of San Francisco in an all-out war on rats is told with humor and pardonable pride in the 1909 *Report of the Citizens' Health Committee.*[9] "Before San Francisco could get rid of plague," the report admits, "it had to go to school and study zoology, bacteriology, and fleas." "Dr. Blue's brigade" had a platoon for every segment of the population, from the Bar Association and the Ship Owners' Association to the San Francisco Labor Council and the Thursday Afternoon Club of the Mission. The work began in September 1907, and the last of 89 cases occurred in January, 1908. In the first six weeks alone, 72,460 premises were inspected, 171 dangerous houses destroyed, and 56,994 rats trapped or found dead. The thoroughness of the work is astonishing. Fear, engendered by the recent natural catastrophe, must have spurred the citizens on. Two years after the alarm was sounded, the Citizens' Health Committee reported to the Mayor that San Francisco had made a new record in sanitation and that the plague had ceased and no trace of it could be found on the peninsula. Dr. Blue departed after a grand farewell banquet at the Fairmont Hotel.

Developed countries have now essentially eliminated the diseases that swept through our major cities until a century ago: plague, cholera, typhus, smallpox, malaria, and yellow fever. Infantile dysentery, scarlet fever, and diphtheria, the great killers of infants and young children, are now mercifully rare. Most of these acute infectious diseases have been controlled by planned action based on a more or less accurate understanding of causation.

The achievements of Drs. Smith and Blue are important, but much more could be written to show how careful observation, planned action, hard work, and a little luck on the part of many others have been instrumental in bringing about our present state of health. This emphasis is necessary because some recent writers, notably René Dubos, have stressed that endemic and epidemic diseases fluctuate in response to influences beyond our control. Dr. Dubos sees much of our present good health as incidental to general social development: "The most effective techniques to avoid disease came out of the attempts to correct by social measures the injustices and the ugliness brought about by industrialization." "The nineteenth-century reformers," he continues, "had immense practical achievements to their credit, but the science of which they boasted was usually made up of catchwords."[10] That judgment seems harsh indeed. Would the sewers have been built, the water supplies protected and inspected, and the buildings ratproofed were it not for the Dr. Smiths and the Dr. Blues organizing, prodding, and guiding the citizens and always putting them to school to the scientific evidence?

Dr. William Osler was moved to uncharacteristic anger during a 1902 civic meeting on the subject of tuberculosis. Addressing the mayor of Baltimore, he exclaimed

> We are sick to death of mayors and first branches and second branches. In heaven's name, what have they done for us in the past? . . . Give us a couple or three good men and true who will run the city as a business corporation. It would not take us a year then, Mr. Mayor, not a year, to get a start on a sewerage system and an infectious-disease hospital, and everything else that the public welfare demands.[11]

Dr. William T. Sedgwick, who was responsible for the application of the new bacteriological knowledge to the purification of water in Massachusetts, wrote a textbook in 1902 entitled *Principles of Sanitary Science and the Public Health.* In his view, several major communicable diseases were by that date "well understood and capable of being scientifically dealt with."[12] The means of control he considered as a form of engineering, which he defined as the "scientific control of the forces and materials of nature for the benefit of man." His book is filled with detailed accounts of how meticulous epidemiological study of specific outbreaks of typhoid and other disease led to their control and the saving of hundreds of lives and millions of dollars.

The battle against infectious disease, which has been fought with much skill, science, and success, is not over. Contrary to what the citizens of San Francisco thought when they toasted Dr. Blue's departure, plague had not been eradicated. We now know that it lingers in the ground squirrels and other small mammals of the western United States. From this reservoir it could again pass into an urban rat population; sporadic cases still do occur, mainly in rural areas.[13]

A more serious and immediate problem for American cities is that some of the diseases anciently associated with crowded cities still exact a significant toll of health and lives, and a few threaten to break through all the barriers yet devised by sanitary science.

URBAN INFECTIONS TODAY

Pneumonia, tuberculosis of the lungs, and syphilis are old urban plagues that persist in modern cities. All three continue to show higher mortality in metropolitan counties than elsewhere, though the lowest rates occur in suburban counties;[14] (see also Fig. 1.2). The probable explanation for this distribution varies for each disease.

The clinical pictures of all three of these diseases have changed since the advent of antibiotics. Pneumonia in the child and young adult can usually be aborted before it reaches the full-blown lobar stage with its life-threatening crisis so familiar to the physicians and the popular literature readers of the nineteenth century. Now, pneumonia is mainly a complication, often a terminal one, in the long course of a chronic illness, such as emphysema, heart failure, or cancer. Since many of these primary conditions are urban associated, it is not surprising to find the same geographic distribution for their major complications.

Tuberculosis is a unique and complex disease, the object of great medical and social interest for centuries.[15] The crowding together of new factory workers in cities in the early days of the Industrial Revolution favored the transmission of tuberculosis by means of the inhalation of infected dust or droplets or by the contamination of food or utensils in taverns and common kitchens.[16] Bovine tuberculosis spread, as milk came to be distributed more widely from larger herds.

A long decline in mortality from tuberculosis, continuing to the present, began in the early nineteenth century, about 50 years before the bacterial cause of the disease was identified and 100 years before any specific therapy was introduced. This apparent lack of relationship between the understanding of the disease and its control has been cited as evidence that general social progress has more to do with the control of infectious disease than had sanitary reform. Since this disease can be transmitted by air as well as in food, and through other animals as well as directly between humans, its epidemiology was not as evident as that of cholera, plague, or typhoid, and it is more difficult to show that measures adopted before the disease was well understood were really effective. Nevertheless, informed and concerned physicians took action as early as knowledge made it possible, and such leaders clearly had an effect on general programs of civic improvement. Dr. Lemuel Shattuck, for example, proposed a plan in 1850 for public health in Massachusetts that included a register of cases of tuberculosis and led to the creation of the first State Board of Health the next year. Dr. Herman Biggs devised a detailed plan to prevent the transmission of tuberculosis in the hospitals of New York City in 1889, only seven years after Koch described the tubercle bacillus, and it would be hard to improve on that plan today, except for the use of antibiotics. The fact that we have been unable to eliminate this disease from any city or state 30 years after the introduction of specific therapy testifies to its stubbornness and suggests that some of the early measures may have been neither more nor less effective than some modern practices.

City dwellers, even today, continue to be exposed to tuberculosis more frequently than people who live eleswhere. Recruits from urban areas during World War II were found to have almost twice as high a positive tuberculin reaction rate as recruits from farm counties.[17] Within central city counties, the new active case rate for tuberculosis varies widely. It is highly correlated with poverty and may be five or six times higher in the poor sections of the city than in the wealthy residential districts.[18] Thus, tuberculosis persists as an urban disease, though the prevalence has now dropped to the point at which mass X-ray screening can no longer be justified.

The venereal diseases, like many other infectious diseases, appeared to be approaching extinction in the mid 1950's under the impact of antibiotics, but their frequency has since risen alarmingly (Fig. 2.3).

Though the data shown are for the United States as a whole, it is probable that most of this increase has occurred in cities. Draftees from urban areas during World War II, for example, were found to have higher rates of positive serological tests for syphilis than draftees from rural areas,[19] though the National Health Examination Survey has not confirmed differences related to residence.[20] Survey data tell more than do rates of reported disease, since reporting is certainly not complete.[21] Cases of syphilis (primary, secondary, and all stages) are reported from 61 major cities of the United States at three times the rate reported from the rest of the country. The gonorrhea rate is almost five times higher in cities than elsewhere.[22] The city, as Meier observes, is a "transaction-maximizing system."[23]

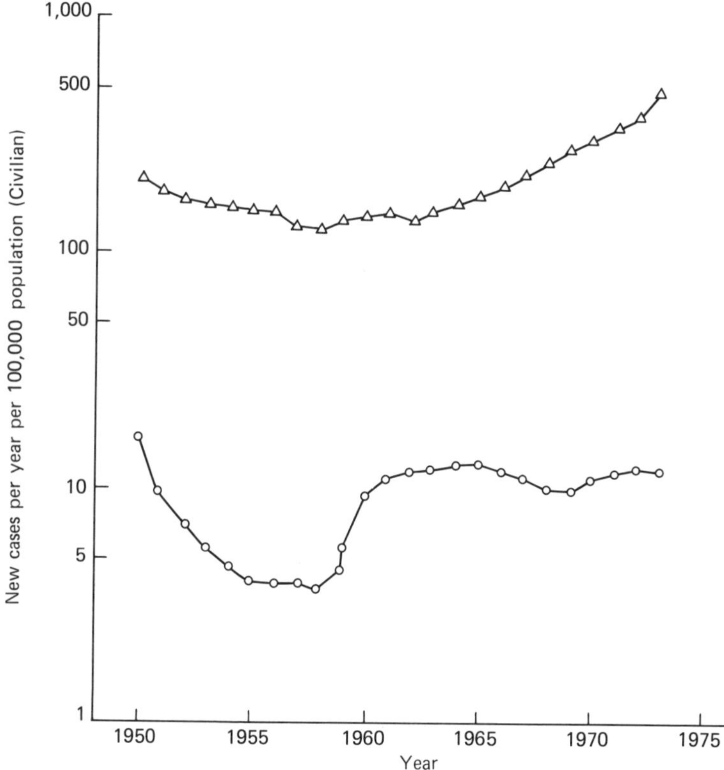

Fig. 2.3 **Gonorrhea** (△) **and primary and secondary syphilis** (○): reported new case rates (U.S.), 1950–1974. Source: U.S. Public Health Service, *Morbidity and Mortality Weekly Report.*

Reasons for the persistence of pneumonia and tuberculosis and for the recent rise in venereal disease are too complex to explore here. Most of the old urban plagues—typhoid, cholera, smallpox, yellow fever, diphtheria—have dropped to inconsequential levels. A few infectious diseases, however, such as bacillary dysentery and measles, do continue as minor causes of death, and their distribution is paradoxical. Proportionately, more cases apparently occur in metropolitan populations, though mortality from these same diseases is reported to be lower in metropolitan counties.[24]

Does this inconsistency reflect more complete reporting in urban counties, do differences in access to treatment reduce metropolitan mortality rates, or do both factors operate?

More accurate differential diagnosis of infectious disease in metropolitan counties may be a factor. Whereas mortality from septicemia, for example, is reported to be slightly higher outside metropolitan counties, deaths from specific types of this infection (streptococcal, staphylococcal, and pneumococcal) are reported more frequently in metropolitan counties, with the unspecified types predominating in non-metropolitan areas.[25]

The significance of infectious diseases in the modern city can be measured in terms of the disability they cause. The National Health Survey reports that farm residents have fewer acute illnesses and related bed disability than do residents of towns or cities, and the picture has been consistent over the nine years for which data are available (Fig. 2.4). Likewise, the influenza epidemic of 1968-1969 apparently resulted in more disability in the cities than on the farms. Such a distribution suggests a more extensive spread of a highly infectious disease under crowded living conditions.

Among the acute diseases reported in these surveys, infectious, parasitic, and upper respiratory diseases show the greatest differences by place of residence. Though such illnesses are more common among children, and there are more children in metropolitan areas, the residential differences for acute conditions are scarcely altered by age-adjustment.[26]

On the whole, the patterns of mortality, morbidity, and disability from acute infectious diseases suggest that the chance of infection is greater in cities than elsewhere and that chronic infections, such as undetected syphilis and tuberculosis, remain major urban health problems.

The lowest mortality rates for infectious disease to be found in the United States are those of the metropolitan non-central city, or suburban counties. This is true for the chronic and persistent diseases, such as tuberculosis and syphilis, as well as for those diseases in which mortality has dropped to almost insignificant levels, for example, scarlet fever, diphtheria, and meningococcal infections. These favorable suburban rates, as we shall see in

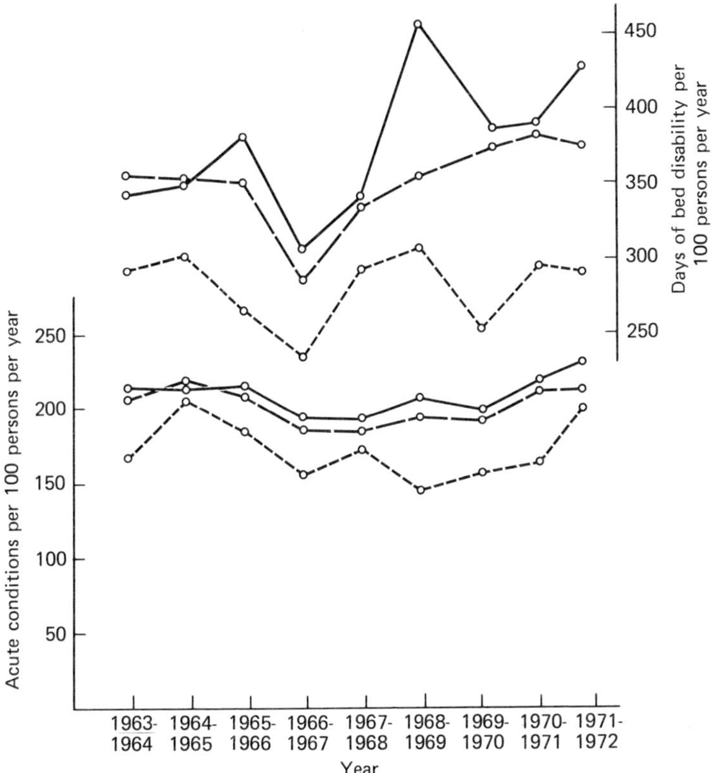

Fig. 2.4 **Incidence of acute conditions and days of bed disability by residence:** (U.S.), 1963–1972. **Key:** SMSA (•—•), non-farm (•— — —•), farm (• - - - •). Source: U.S. National Center for Health Statistics, *Vital and Health Statistics, Series 10.*

Chapter 6, probably reflect better access to and use of diagnostic and treatment services.

ERADICATING INFECTIOUS DISEASE

Action directed at eliminating infectious disease from the busy and crowded cities of the United States over the past 150 years has been successful beyond the dreams of the early reformers, and the consequences of this great experiment extend far into the future. Sanitation and the public health services of American cities have been instrumental in reducing death and disease from water-borne and other infectious diseases to the present low levels.[27] There is a reasonable certainty of completely eliminating smallpox from the face of the globe.[28] We can be proud of what has been done and confident that present urban health problems will also prove to have rational solutions.

But there are also reasons for caution and humility. Dubos wisely reminds us that man has always dreamed of a Golden Age, whether in the past or the future, and he predicts that perfect health will continue to be a mirage.[29] The plague still lies in wait, syphilis is on the rise again, poliomyelitis recurs when we neglect immunization, and increasing numbers of citizens who have never had contact with such diseases as typhoid or cholera would be highly susceptible should a natural or man-made catastrophe disrupt our carefully constructed defenses. We cannot afford to forget an old and honored objective of urban health: freedom from serious infectious disease.

The first requirement is to maintain a vigilant defense. The United States Public Health Service collects information, conducts research, and initiates nation-wide epidemic control measures at the Center for Disease Control in Atlanta, Georgia. In describing the program to a British audience in 1970, Dr. Alexander Langmuir, then the director, cited some impressive examples of its effectiveness but also admitted, "The methods of surveillance are intrinsically crude and inaccurate. Reporting of cases is usually incomplete, verification of diagnosis is often lacking or delayed, adequacy of follow up of significant cases varies, and death registration, at least in the U.S.A., is cumbersome."[30]

Better technology and engineering are needed here, as in the control of damaging effects of the physical environment. More efficient information systems, immunization against venereal and other diseases, cheaper and more reliable methods of disease detection–there is a great deal of scientific work cut out for us. As we come to be bound closer to the rest of the world by satellites and jet planes, it is increasingly clear that, in our own self-interest, we must export to developing countries not arms and armies, but vaccines, antibiotics, and public health experts who can work with physicians and other leaders toward the world-wide control of disease. The time is ripe for a revitalization of public health, and some socialist countries, such as China and Cuba, have recognized the potential of this revitalization very clearly.[31, 32]

There is also much to be done on the social action front here at home. One encouraging study indicates that four inner-city comprehensive-care programs in Baltimore, by the systematic finding and treatment of streptococcal infections among urban children, have succeeded in reducing the incidence of rheumatic fever.[33] This is important evidence that organized efforts to furnish good health care to an underserved central city population will improve health measurably. Increased application of the skills and knowledge we already possess will, in all probability, extend our control over other infectious diseases.[34] Can we guarantee all our children the protection of proven methods of immunization, with due regard for personal rights? How many American teenagers today know the basic facts about the transmission and prevention of venereal disease? How many state or national legislators have even a rudimentary understanding of the relationship between waste disposal and human health or between good vital statistics and the control of tuberculosis?

Sir MacFarlane Burnet put the social issue clearly in the introduction to his *Natural History of Infectious Disease:* "We can never forget that the apparent impotence of infectious disease over most of the world depends wholly on the maintenance of the structure of civilization and the intelligent and continuing application of the discoveries of the past."[35]

The control of disease arising from the physical environment and from infections, though challenging and complex, is practicable because it can be based on increasingly solid scientific fact. In contrast, injury, disease, and death that originate in the social environment of the modern city are less well understood and therefore, more difficult to measure and regulate. In the next two chapters, we will consider how new patterns and pressures of urban life affect the health of the citizens, particularly those who are most vulnerable: the children, the aged, the disabled, and the chronically ill.

3 A DANGEROUS PLACE TO GROW UP

"The United States was born in the country and has moved to the city." In this terse summary of our social history, Richard Hofstadter suggests the source of many of our contemporary problems of urban health.[1] Whether the settlers of American cities came from the farms and villages of Europe or from our own rural countryside, they brought with them the habits and culture of simpler, more even-paced lives. In contrast with cherished memories of the ancestral village or the old family farm, crowded city streets and raucous factories seemed to threaten body and mind.

MAN AND THE MACHINE

The new industrial cities of the nineteenth century were indeed dangerous places, and the dangers arose from the exploitation of human labor and from uncompensated industrial injuries as well as from crowding and "filth diseases."

The United States, however, had been spared the worst abuses of the early industrial revolution. In England, according to official reports, children were once sold to mill owners for five pounds apiece, and women were harnessed like horses to coal trucks in the mines. The English Factory Act of 1833, the first effective industrial legislation, restricted the working hours of children between the ages of 9 and 18 to 12 hours a day and 69 a week.[2] Child labor laws and the regulation of working conditions and hours were gradually achieved in England by the work of courageous reformers of the eighteenth and early nineteenth centuries. The employer's responsibility to compensate the worker for industrial accidents, however, was not clearly established in that country until 1897, though it had been recognized 50 years earlier in Austria and other European countries.[3]

In the United States, industry started later, and the stream of cheap immigrant labor during the rapid expansion of the middle and late nineteenth century provided a compliant and fluid work force. Reform came late as well. In 1886, the State of New York finally passed a law regulating the employment of women and children in manufacturing establishments and providing for inspection. Two inspectors were appointed, and their *First Report* gives glimpses of the health risks faced by factory workers in cities of the United States less than 100 years ago.[4]

The inspectors estimated that about 8,000 children under the age of 13 had been excluded from factory work by the new law. Before it was passed, they stated, "it was not uncommon for children seven or eight years old to be seen trudging before daylight to the factory, and after twelve hours of steady work and confinement, trudging back to their homes after dark." Many factory buildings were found to be unsafe and unsanitary: "It is a rule in many factories visited by us to keep the doors locked. The key is usually kept in the pocket of the foreman or porter." Heavy machinery was unguarded: "The machines used for stamping metal are extremely dangerous, and boys and girls are chiefly employed on them. One day, in the office of a factory, the Inspector met a boy looking for work who had lost two fingers where previously employed. When asked why he didn't return to work where he was injured, he said that the loss of his fingers made him useless to his former employer."

Jacob Riis, Danish immigrant, journalist, companion of Theodore Roosevelt when he was Police President of New York City, and passionate reformer, touched the conscience of his adopted countrymen with his book *How the Other Half Lives* in 1890. He went where the factory inspectors were not authorized to go, into the busy shops and the teeming tenements of the East Side.[5] There he found masses of recent immigrants, "herded in great numbers in the so-called tenement factories, where the cheapest grade of work is done at the lowest wages." "Up two flights of dark stairs, three, four, with new smells of cabbage, of onion, of frying fish, on every landing, whirring sewing machines behind closed doors betraying what goes on within." In one room he found, "five men and a woman, two young girls, not fifteen, and a boy who says unasked that he is fifteen, and lies in saying it, are at the machines sewing knickerbockers. . . . They turn out one hundred and twenty dozen 'knee-pants' a week, for which the manufacturer pays seventy cents a dozen."

Saleswomen, Riis reported

> receiving $1.75 a week for work that at certain seasons lengthened their days to sixteen hours, were sometimes required to pay for their aprons. On account of the oppressive heat and lack of ventilation, "girls fainted day after day and came out looking like corpses;" a common cause for discharge from employment was "too long service." No other fault was found with the discharged saleswomen than that they had been long enough in the employ of the firm to justly expect an increase of salary. The reason was given with brutal frankness, in some instances.

In 1910, according to a report to the Senate, 20 percent of the men employed in blast furnaces and steel mills worked 84 hours or more per week, which meant a 12-hour working day every day of the week.[6]

When Alice Hamilton, a physician working with immigrants at Hull House in Chicago in 1910, became concerned about the health and safety of industrial workers, she found a total lack of interest and knowledge among her medical friends.[7] A workmen's compensation law was passed in 1916, in part, as a result of her work and of pressure from the American labor movement. The field of industrial medicine at last began to take form, and the collection of statistics was started. It was not until 1948 that workmen's compensation became nationwide, with the enactment of a law in Mississippi.[8]

Even though we have only meager data to document the changes, there has clearly been important progress in occupational safety. Disabling work injuries in manufacturing occurred at the rate of 23 per million man-hours worked in 1926-1928 and had been reduced to 15.2 by 1970.

"Dangerous trades," as Dr. Hamilton called them, remain dangerous, however, as indicated by the fact that the rate of injury in coal mining has been reduced only from about 80 to 40 per million man-hours worked in the past 40 years. This figure may be compared with low rates in such occupations as banking (2 injuries per million man-hours) and civil service jobs (6-7 per million man-hours).[9, 10] If we had the data that would enable us to look back over a span of 100 years or more, as we can with reports of infectious diseases, we would probably find very large reductions in death and injury related to work.

The successes of occupational health reforms, like those of sanitation, have had the curious effect of creating a new environment in which it is easy to forget the cruel hours and dangerous conditions under which our forebears worked. Now, in order to perceive that urban working conditions are relatively safe, we must compare them with conditions on the farm, where unregulated safety hazards and child labor are still to be found.[11]

Accident mortality and work-related injuries are less common today among city dwellers than among individuals who live outside metropolitan areas. The risk of dying in an accident is considerably lower for city dwellers (Fig. 3.1). Central cities and suburbs have similar rates in this respect, and the rates for both are lower than non-metropolitan rates by approximately one-third. The higher rural death rates for motor vehicle accidents can be explained by the fact that traffic accidents, which are more frequent in the city, occur at lower speeds there and tend to produce injuries, whereas rural accidents have a much higher case fatality rate (1:10.5, compared with 1:250 for urban accidents).[12] Ironically, the urban traffic jam may save lives by reducing speed.

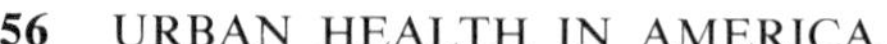

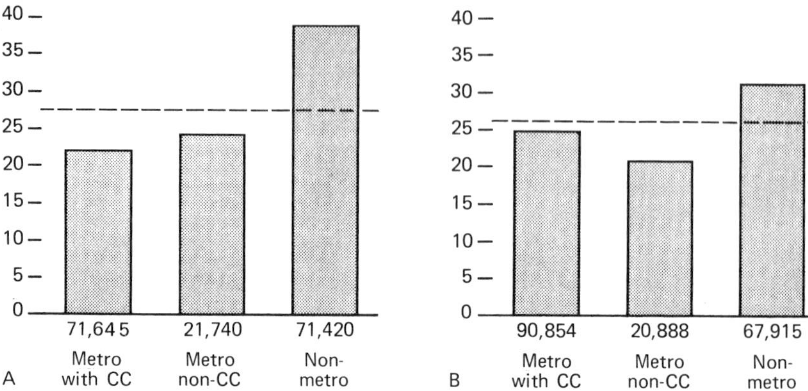

Fig. 3.1 **Deaths attributed to** (A) **motor vehicle accidents** (ICDA E810-E823) **and** (B) **all other accidents** (ICDA E800-E807, E825-E949): age-adjusted annual mortality rates (U.S.), 1969–1971, by county of residence. (Cf. Fig. 1.1 and Appendix B, Tables 25 and 26.)

Non-fatal, work-related injuries, as well as accidental deaths, occur at lower rates in metropolitan areas. This difference suggests that safety practices are better organized and better observed in factories than they are on farms, where the rates of such injuries are 49 percent higher.[13] On farms, injury rates of all kinds are relatively higher among older persons, being 30 percent higher than in metropolitan areas for those over the age of 45.[14]

Though the dangers of physical injury at work have been greatly reduced over several decades, a significant number of injuries continue to occur, and that number may be increasing slightly. Among male blue-collar workers in metropolitan areas in the year 1966-1967, 28.5 percent sustained injuries at work that required medical attention or restricted activity for a day or more. In manufacturing, the rate of disabling work injuries increased between 1960 and 1970 from 12.0 to 15.2 per million man-hours worked.[15] Nationwide, the average annual rate of work-related injuries per 100 employed persons has risen from 12.3 in 1961-1963 to 13.8 in 1966-1967.[16]

New kinds of industrial health hazards are constantly being introduced with the production of new chemicals the toxic effects of which are poorly understood.[17] The mining, processing, and use of radioactive materials also introduces unmeasured health risks to local populations, due to an increased low-level radiation in the environment, and poses the unsolved dilemma of how to store waste products that will remain dangerous for hundreds of years.[18] Thus, new hazards for the industrial worker are continually being added to such recognized and partially controlled hazards as mechanical injury by heavy machinery and cancer produced by chromates, asbestos, and other substances. Knowledge, interest, and resources in the field of occupational health appear once more to be falling behind the expansion and increasing complexity of modern industry.

The worker's health is also threatened by changing circumstances in an entirely different quarter. Ironically, the reduction of the physical risks of work exposes an underlying psychological problem first identified by such nineteenth-century analysts of the industrial revolution as de Tocqueville, Marx, and Weber. The alienation of the worker from his work may ultimately prove to be more dangerous than industrial accidents and long hours. A 1973 report to the Department of Health, Education and Welfare finds that "dull repetitive, seemingly meaningless tasks, offering little challenge or autonomy, are causing discontent among workers at all occupational levels. This is not so much because work itself has greatly changed; indeed, one of the main problems is that work has not changed fast enough to keep up with the rapid and widespread changes in worker attitudes, aspirations and values."[19]

There is increasing concern about the "blue collar blues," and at least one study finds that the assembly-line worker in an automotive plant tends to regard both himself and his job with contempt and to seek his life-satisfactions away from work.[20] In metropolitan areas, workers report an average of 5.4 days lost from work per year, compared to 4.8 for those employed on farms.[21] Moreover, employers report to the Labor Department that persons with a job but not at work at any given time rose from 4.1 percent in 1950 to 6.1 percent in 1974, the increases being attributed mainly to "illness" and longer vacations.[22]

CITY LIFE

The streets, homes, and public places of American cities are likely to be even more dangerous than the work places. Large concentrations of population provide a ready market for alcohol and other drugs, and subculture customs and the stress of urban life encourage their use. A fast pace of living and anonymity facilitate casual sexual encounters, with the predictable consequences of illegitimacy, abortion, and venereal disease. Homicide and rape have increased alarmingly. But the most serious threat to human health and life in the modern American city is probably the whole vicious cycle of poverty, with its heavy impact on children and young adults.

Though work may be safer in the city than elsewhere, other kinds of activities are not. Non-work injuries are more common in metropolitan than in non-metropolitan areas. These include traffic injuries and injuries at home and in "other places."[13, 23]

Like acute infectious diseases, injuries appear to be a special danger for young people living in densely populated areas. Below the age of 45, the average number of injuries is 20 percent higher for metropolitan residents than for farm residents, whereas above 45, the relationships are exactly reversed.[14] The same pattern is reported for general disability (acute and chronic) among younger people, whether measured by days of restricted activity, days of bed disability, or days lost from school.[24, 25]

Some injuries result from violent crime, and the recent rise in urban homicide will be considered below. Relatively high rates of injury among young people in the city are probably also related to the use of automobiles and to such social factors as crowding and unsafe housing. The higher rates of disability among urban youth also have multiple causes. Injury is one, and a higher incidence of infectious disease is another. Though chronic disability is generally more prevalent outside cities, more young metropolitan residents report that they have one or more chronic conditions than do young people elsewhere,[24, 26] and the rates are even higher among young people (under 17) in areas of urban poverty, such as those selected as sites for neighborhood health centers.[27]

Addiction

One such chronic condition may well be alcoholism and its complications. Fatal cirrhosis of the liver shows a more dramatic correlation with urbanization than any other cause of death, and the rate in central city counties is nearly twice that in non-metropolitan counties (Fig. 3.2). Extrapolating from the fact that one-half the men who die of cirrhosis have been diagnosed as alcoholics,

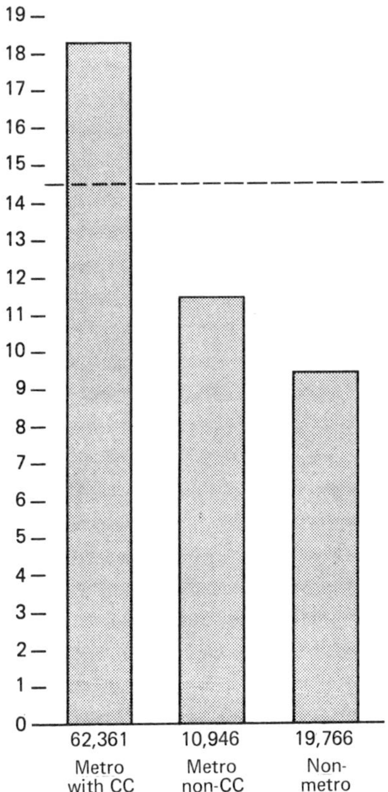

Fig. 3.2 **Deaths attributed to cirrhosis of liver** (ICDA 571): age-adjusted annual mortality rates (U.S.), 1969–1971, by county of residence. (Cf. Fig. 1.1 and Appendix B, Table 21.)

one can estimate that there are 6 million alcoholics in the United States.[28] Alcoholism is undoubtedly a major health problem in this country. A nationwide interview survey of American drinking practices in 1964-1965 gave the first uniform information on this subject. The proportion of persons who said they drink at least once a year ranges from 43 percent among farm residents to 87 percent among those living in the largest suburbs. Large central cities have the highest proportion of residents who are heavy drinkers (22 to 23 percent) or who admit that they drink to escape life's problems (10 to 12 percent). Large cities and suburbs also have high proportions of individuals who drink maximum amounts. Drinkers, therefore, are most frequently found at the country club and the suburban cocktail party, but heavy drinkers are most numerous in the corner tavern.[29]

A special urban type of alcoholic is the social "loser" who gravitates to the skid-row section of the inner city where cheap liquor, food, and shelter can be obtained and where misery can find company.[30] Alcoholism, like many other city health problems, is closely related to poverty and all its secondary effects.

Though the abuse of alcohol is widespread, with definite urban concentrations, drug addiction is almost entirely an urban phenomenon. Well over one-half the known opiate addicts in the United States live in New York, Chicago, or Los Angeles. Within large cities, addicts are concentrated in deteriorating neighborhoods and slum ghettos. Somewhat surprisingly, the use of drugs (apart from alcohol) is not prevalent in skid-row areas.

Most addicts in the United States are young adults—50 percent under the age of 30 and 80 percent under 40—and the peak age of first opiate use is 16 to 17 years. A marked change has taken place in the addict population in the past 30 years. The proportion of non-whites among addicts admitted to the national hospital in Lexington, Kentucky, has risen from 11.6 to 56 percent; and increases are greatest for the black and Spanish-speaking population of northern cities.[31]

Because drug addiction is both illegal and socially disapproved of in our general culture, it is difficult to be sure how prevalent it is. A review of the long history of opiate addiction in the United

States suggests, surprisingly, that there has been a marked decrease over the past 50 years.[32] Contrary to this long-term trend, "epidemic" waves of heroin addiction have very recently been described in Washington, D.C.[33] and Chicago.[34] The rate of increase seems to be particularly high in New York City, where, as in other large cities, the use of heroin is radiating out of mainly black ghetto areas into white middle-class schools and neighborhoods.[35] Narcotics addiction and its complications have become the leading cause of death for young people (ages 15 to 35) in New York City.[36]

Drug addiction has social causes and social effects. Ball and Chambers, in a comprehensive study of the epidemiology of opiate addiction in the United States, point out, "In many respects opiate addiction is similar to both juvenile delinquency and venereal disease. As with delinquency it is a peer-group phenomenon pursued in a recreational or street setting. As with venereal disease it is commonly transmitted by personal contacts which are intentional."[37] Despite the hidden nature of addiction, it is clear that the use of heroin in our cities is linked to an enormously profitable international opium traffic[38] and that the need to maintain a habit, which may cost $75 to $100 a day, leads to increased crimes against person and property.[39]

Abortion and illegitimacy

The same city streets that foster drug addiction also offer multitudinous occasions for sex. The recent rise in venereal disease was described in the last chapter. Illegitimacy and abortion are additional health problems with strong social components, which appear to be concentrated in cities. A sweeping increase in the legalization and open practice of abortion is under way in Western countries.[40] The Supreme Court has invalidated laws restricting a woman's access to abortion in the first three months of pregnancy, and key public opinion on the subject is rapidly changing.[41, 42] Because of legal and social taboos, no satisfactory information about the incidence of abortion in cities of the United States has been available in the past. With the advent of legal abortion, however, early reports indicate that abortion deaths and complications are declining and infant health improving. Urban and suburban women will evidently be the first to make use of the service.

Maternal mortality rates are generally lower in cities than in rural areas. A striking exception, however, is death from septic abortion, which has been more frequent in cities than elsewhere. This pattern is consistently found among whites and others and in all regions of the country.[43] These data are from 1960, and do not reflect recent changes. The legalization of abortion in New York State has been followed by a sharp drop in maternal mortality rates.[44] Though it is still too early to be certain of the fact, it looks as though a long-standing urban threat to health, the untrained or illegal abortionist, may yield to altered social structures and attitudes as he never yielded to punitive laws.

The number of illegitimate births per 1,000 unmarried women 15 to 44 years of age has risen significantly in the United States over the past 30 years.[45, 46] Metropolitan rates have been 20 percent higher than the rates in non-metropolitan counties. Though illegitimacy may seem to be more a social problem than a medical one, it is closely related to health. Illegitimate babies have in the past been more likely to be underweight and to be delivered at home and by midwives, and illegitimate pregnancy is more likely to end in fetal death. But these dangers are also mainly those of rural childbirth. Non-white rates of illegitimate birth have long been higher than the rates for white women by a factor of ten or more. Non-white rates, however, have leveled off in the past 10 years, whereas white rates have continued to rise. We are seeing an important change in social attitudes toward illegitimacy, as well as toward abortion, related to the women's liberation movement and the counter-culture life style of young people. Even now, it is not so unusual, as it was until very recently in this country, for an unmarried woman to choose to bear a child.[47] The number of families in metropolitan areas headed by a man increased about 13 percent between 1960 and 1970, while families headed by a woman increased about 40 percent.[48] Some of the rise in illegitimacy rates is probably elective rather than accidental. If illegitimacy becomes socially acceptable, as is abortion in many circles now, many aspects of urban life may change, and childbirth could become safer.

Homicide

Homicide is the classic crime of violence. Recent assassinations and the dramatic increase in homicide rates for many cities give the impression that it is an urban phenomenon. In fact, like poverty, homicide occurs at relatively high and increasing rates in city slums and in depressed agricultural areas (Fig. 3.3). As the most extreme act of social and interpersonal conflict, homicide

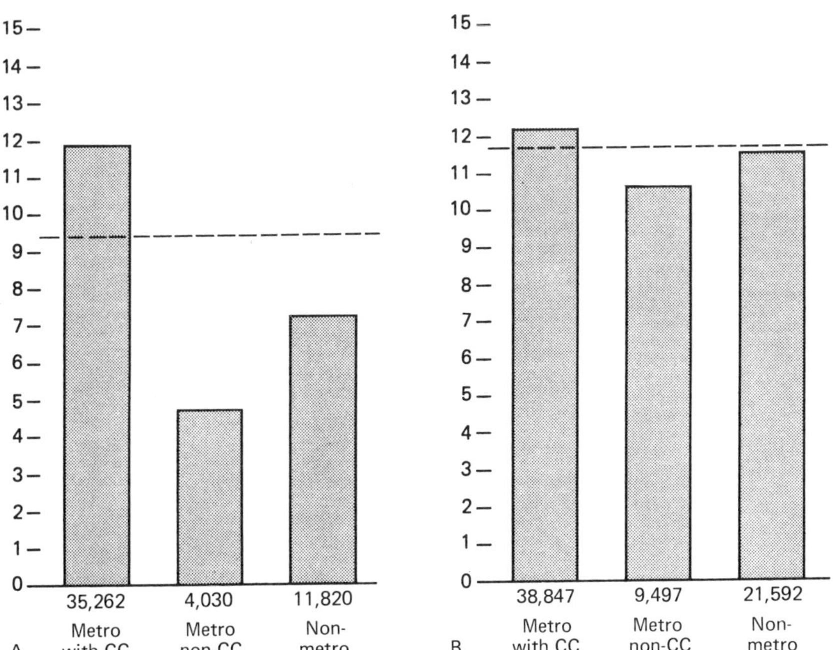

Fig. 3.3 **Deaths attributed to** (A) **homicide** (ICDA E960-E978) **and** (B) **suicide** (ICDA E950-E959): age-adjusted annual mortality rates (U.S.), 1969–1971, by county of residence. (Cf. Fig. 1.1 and Appendix B, Tables 27 and 28.)

may be a more direct indicator of social stress than is suicide, which Durkheim examined in his classic sociological study of 1897.[49] Among measures of health status, homicide is one of the most objective and specific. It is probably the least equivocal cause of death, and by its nature as well as by law it is highly likely to be recorded.

Several studies of homicide in cities of the United States have been made, based on the records of Birmingham,[50] Houston,[51] Philadelphia,[52] and Cleveland.[53, 54] Homicide has repeatedly been shown in these studies to occur at higher rates in poor sections of the cities and to be associated with crowding, bad housing, other slum conditions, and unemployment. As for the personal characteristics of those individuals involved in the crime, most studies deal with information about the victim, rather than the assailant, since it is usually more readily available and complete. Victims and assailants resemble each other, however, since all these studies show that murder usually occurs between two persons who are closely connected by ties of family, marriage, sex, or intimate association. Both victims and assailants are overwhelmingly young adult, male, poor, and non-white.

In addition, much urban in-migration of the past two decades has been shown to originate in non-metropolitan areas, with high homicide rates, where there has been a demonstrable tradition of violence.[55, 56] These observations, reinforced by less well documented impressions, have led some to suggest that "many homicides were committed by recent Negro migrants from the South"[57] or that "the violent crime rate of Negroes who have moved from the South into the large urban cities is far higher than the national crime rate for Negroes."[58] The implication that poor black people from the rural south or poor white people from the Appalachian hills are responsible for urban crime and violence is unproven. Some evidence, in fact, indicates that migrants are less likely than established residents to participate in such forms of urban violence as delinquency or rioting.[59] Two different hypotheses could explain the two peaks of homicide rates in urban and rural areas: (a) urban homicide is an expression of a "culture of violence" transmitted from poor rural areas to large industrial cities by extensive in-migration over the past 20 years; and (b) urban homicide results from social stress produced by this same migration, particularly when housing, employment, and services are inadequate to meet the needs of the in-migrants.

The wave of urban violence in the late 1960's was accompanied by a sharp and sustained rise in homicide rates in major cities of the United States.[54] Concern over this increase in overt social violence has forced us to re-examine other possible explanations. Wolfgang has assembled an impressive list of factors associated with urban homicide: poverty, physical deterioration of the environment, low educational levels, residence in industrial or commercial centers, unemployed or unskilled labor status, economic dependency, marital instability, lack of male role models, overcrowding, lack of opportunity, absence of anticriminal behavior patterns, more organic disease, and subcultural or minority status.[60] Taken together, these factors, each with some plausible causal relationship to the crime, show homicide to be an index of powerful cultural and interpersonal stress in our urban society. Even more persons are directly affected by violence than is indicated by the homicide figures. For every fatal attack, there are some six aggravated assaults known to police and an unknown number of unreported conflicts that lead to injury and disability.[61]

URBAN POVERTY AND ILL HEALTH

> To live in Harlem is to dwell in the very bowels of the city; it is to pass a labyrinthine existence among streets that explode monotonously skyward with the spires and crosses of churches and clutter under foot with garbage and decay. Harlem is a ruin —many of its ordinary aspects (its crimes, its casual violence, its crumbling buildings with littered areaways, ill-smelling halls and vermin-invaded rooms) are indistinguishable from the distorted images that appear in dreams, and which, like muggers haunting a lonely hall, quiver in the waking mind with hidden and threatening significance. Yet this is no dream but the reality of well over four hundred thousand Americans; a reality which for many defines and colors the world. Overcrowded and exploited politically and economically, Harlem is the scene and symbol of the Negro's perpetual alienation in the land of his birth.[62]

Ralph Ellison's grim portrait of one segment of the inner city can be documented, though the poverty of many central city residents and the ill health that accompanies it can also be hidden from view by statistical generalizations as well as by geographic segregation. Average rates of infant and maternal mortality, for example, are reported in one major study as being lower in urban than in rural counties.[43] In fact, poor infants and mothers are more likely to die than are those in households with better resources, and a great many poor people are concentrated in large city slums. Certain parts of the city, on closer examination, prove to have grossly excessive infant and maternal mortality rates, though these rates in the city as a whole are actually lower than the rates in non-urban areas.

The inner city

Sixteen areas of New York City with low incomes were compared with the rest of the city over a three-year period (1961-1963). Excesses in the poor sections ranged from 55 to 299 percent in terms of infant and maternal mortality, proportion of mothers registering late in pregnancy, premature births, illegitimacy rates, cases of syphilis, and crude death rates from tuberculosis.[63]

A detailed study of infant deaths in New York City in 1968, though it does not examine differences by geographic areas, does bring out clearly the fact that infant mortality within an urban population varies widely relative to social and demographic factors. White, native-born mothers, for example, experienced an infant mortality rate (deaths in the first year of life) of 15.2 per 1,000 live births, compared with 25.4 for mothers born in Puerto Rico and 35.7 for black, native-born mothers. Mothers with an elementary education or none had an infant mortality of 27.7 per 1,000 live births, whereas the figure for those with a year or more of college was only 12.9. Limited education and minority status are measures of social class and imply limited understanding of and resources for coping with the problems of obtaining health care in an urban environment.

In a more recent study of 19 large cities of the United States, health indices were examined in relation to poverty status (by census tracts) and race (Table 3.1). Within these large cities, the

Table 3.1
Vital statistics for an average of 19 large cities of the United States, by income area and color (1969-1971)

	LOW-INCOME AREAS			*REMAINDER OF CITY*		
	Total	*White*	*All Other*	*Total*	*White*	*All Other*
Low birth weight (2,500 grams or less) (per 100 live births)	13.1	9.3	15.1	8.3	7.0	12.4
Infant mortality rate (per 1,000 live births)	30.2	24.2	33.4	19.7	17.4	27.0
No prenatal care (per 100 live births)	5.0	4.2	5.3	1.8	1.5	2.8
Illegitimate births (per 100 live births)	40.8	23.7	49.5	13.1	7.3	30.9
Death rate from tuberculosis (per 100,000 population)	9.5	8.7	10.0	3.0	2.8	4.3
Death rate from violent causes (per 100,000 population)	115.5	112.7	117.1	61.9	59.0	75.7

Source: S. J. Ventura, S. M. Taffel, and E. Spratley, "Vital and health statistics for low-income areas in 19 large cities, 1969-1971" (Paper presented at annual meeting, American Public Health Association, New Orleans, La., Oct. 24, 1974).

low-income areas experienced rates of low birth weight, infant mortality, inadequate prenatal care, illegitimacy, and deaths from tuberculosis and from violent causes that were from one and one-half to more than three times higher than in the higher income areas. A large part of these differences is related to income, but differences related to race also persist, both in the poorer and in the more affluent parts of the cities.[64]

Migration and jobs

When rodents are given a large, protected, open area in which to live, with a uniformly available food supply, abnormal behavior limits the maximum population. This behavior, as observed under more controlled conditions, leads to a remarkable social pattern, which has been called a "behavioral sink." As the population density increases, dominant animals become more aggressive, weaker animals are ostracized, fertility drops, and disease and a variety of forms of social pathology develop.[65]

There are some striking similarities, as well as many differences, between this rodent behavior and the drive of human beings who congregate in cities.[66] The central cities of the United States have always attracted large numbers of migrants, mainly poor people, first from the farms and cities of Europe, and now from our own southern farms and mountains and from Puerto Rico and Cuba. Competition produces winners and losers, aggression and violence exert selective force, and the weak pay a penalty with their health and, sometimes, their lives.

Until recently, the American city has not been a dead-end, like the rodent "sink" but instead has worked reasonably well as a social transmission mechanism for receiving the migrant poor, sheltering them, giving them room to strive and live with others and a chance at education and employment; these opportunities have often opened the way to prosperity and suburban life. Rather suddenly, however, this cycle has changed, and large sections of the inner city seem to have become traps that concentrate poverty. Though both the numbers and the proportions of persons below the poverty level decreased significantly in this country between 1960 and 1970, the proportion of the poor in central city counties increased from 26.9 to 32.0 percent.[48]

The reason for the change is to be found on the output rather than on the intake side of the urban social process. The 1970 census showed that poor people are continuing to migrate to northern cities from the rural south and Appalachian mountains at the same rate as they have over the past 20 years.[67] Figures on the urban drift of the downwardly socially mobile are lacking, but there is no reason to think that the influx of these newly poor people has changed either.

What has happened is that opportunities for education and economic advancement of the urban poor have shrunk. The operative social forces are racial discrimination for many and the disappearance of unskilled jobs and recurrent political, administrative, and economic crises in the functioning of city government for all. Blacks and Puerto Ricans are marked by their skin color, their accents, or both. Along with all the other handicaps associated with membership in a subculture or racial minority, the visible identity of the recent urban migrants has made possible their systematic exclusion from housing, jobs, schools, and other social institutions that were made available to the earlier white European immigrants. Progress has been made toward opening up all of these avenues to minority groups, but many roadblocks remain. Even while the urban poor are spending much of their energy in the struggle to overcome discrimination, they are doubly frustrated by the disappearance of unskilled jobs as a result of increasing mechanization and automation of industry. The shift from manual to skilled jobs effectively removes the first rung of the ladder.[68] The gap between the median family income of central city families and that of suburban families nearly doubled from $930 in 1960 to $1,850 in 1970.[48] On top of these problems, the bankruptcy and near paralysis of many metropolitan governments prevent the modernization and expansion of city schools, hospitals, social, and other services, which have made life tolerable and advancement possible for city dwellers in the past.

These forces are so potent that they have disconnected large segments of the urban poor from the economic system. Moynihan has pointed out that during a period of generally increasing prosperity, the poorest sections of our cities have actually become poorer and that we may be witnessing the development of a "fixed underclass."[69] The most alarming possibility is that of total alienation of a whole segment of society, with segregation into armed and hostile urban and suburban camps. This is the picture drawn in 1969 by the National Commission on the Causes and Prevention of Violence (Eisenhower Commission) as the potential outcome of existing social trends, unless effective public action is taken.[70]

Though such an extreme rift seems unlikely, the fact that a group of prominent citizens considers it possible suggests that social differences, which have been notably fluid in this country in the past, are becoming more rigid.

The cycle of poverty

The geographic distribution of the population coincides in part with its distribution on the social scale. Income is a primary index of status, and social and economic status, in turn, is an important determinant of health. Two groups are particularly vulnerable: those who are born poor, and those who become poor.

The cycle of poverty can be viewed as both a cause and an effect of ill health, since each tends to perpetuate the other.[71] Many of the health disadvantages of urban life cited in previous chapters can be traced to their association with poverty. A baby born to a poor mother, whether on the farm or in an urban ghetto, is more likely to be premature and less likely to survive birth, the first month, or the first year than is a baby born to a more fortunate suburban mother. The former is more likely to be illegitimate and to grow up without a father. In childhood and youth, the poor person has less and poorer education and lives in a culture that is commonly burdened by racial discrimination, crime, personal violence, and unstable sex and family patterns. High rates of venereal disease, mental impairment, homicide and other crimes of violence, drug addiction, and juvenile delinquency form the background of daily life. Individual growth and development are more likely to be retarded than among the more affluent.[72] The environment of urban poverty perpetuates the cycle that begins with the unhealthy conditions surrounding pregnancy.

Poor people in the United States are usually looked down upon and often considered inferior. At the same time, we like to romanticize the lives of poor people, preferably from the vantage point of a successful rise out of threadbare beginnings. "It is easier to praise poverty than to live in it." In spite of the essentially morbid effect of poverty on physical and mental health, life in urban slums does have positive qualities. An element of the culture of poverty so vividly described by Oscar Lewis is a capacity for spontaneity and adventure arising from an orientation to the present and a ready release from frustration by social mechanisms that often involve violence.[73] Poor people in the West End of

Boston, before that area was "renewed," had a sense of neighborhood identity and made life bearable for each other with an expressive life style.[74] Mental health among the urban poor might be worse were it not for such mutual support.

Cities of the United States have some of the worst slums found in the Western world. But they are not completely static slums. Probably no more than 20 percent of those below the poverty level actually share the deprivation and hopelessness of the real culture of poverty–but this still means that 6 to 10 million people do.[73] On the average, until the current recession, the poor had been working their way out of poverty at the rate of more than a million persons a year.[69]

HABITABLE CITIES

Strikes, injuries, homicides, drugs, and unemployment have become such familiar items in the daily news that the shock wears off and resignation sets in. How can a distracted Congress or a fragmented and bankrupt urban government respond adequately? Occupational safety codes are out of date, the welfare system seems to be a failing social experiment, police and courts appear ineffectual or worse, and the individual citizen is moved to look first of all to his own safety. Are there any rational steps to take–any glimmer of hope for a more habitable city?

The effort to achieve a safer and more humane urban life logically begins with defining the objective. Remote though it may seem from present reality, we have the capacity to create a social environment that favors the development of human potential.

Technological and managerial remedies

Part of the solution to the problem of making work less dangerous lies in simply applying what we already know. The evidence that lung disease and cancer can be caused by certain substances used in manufacturing, such as asbestos, chromates, and beryllium, has been slow to accumulate but is now becoming irrefutable.[75] It is imperative that human exposure to these substances be eliminated or rigorously controlled and that the provisions of the

Occupational Safety and Health Act be enforced. A great deal more must be known about whether prolonged exposure of workers to numerous other substances, such as low level radioactivity and a wide range of organic chemicals, can also cause malignant changes and genetic or developmental abnormalities.[76] Successful prosecution of these studies and the use of their findings to protect the worker's health will require the combined forces of governmental research, inspection, and enforcement, enlightened self-interest on the part of employers, and continued alertness and pressure from labor unions.

Work alienation is a more complex problem than that of physical danger, since it arises from deep-seated attitudes toward self and society. The ultimate source of work motivation and job satisfaction is now being recognized as inherent in the performance of the task itself rather than in the physical and social context of the job. Encouraging experiments are being conducted in this country and in Sweden in which assembly-line tasks are being reordered so that the worker can achieve a sense of having produced an identifiable product. Job interest can also be increased when the worker has the largest possible share in making decisions about what he does.[77] Rising work absence rates, strikes provoked by psychological and social conditions of work, and the appearance of new man-machine interrelationships all focus attention on the human characteristics and needs of the worker. The trend toward services as the largest category of employment may increase the intrinsic interest of work, though the danger of bureaucratic boredom is certainly as great as that of monotony on the assembly line. The rationalization, redistribution, and humanization of the work of health care, for example, is an urgent task, which we will examine more closely in Chapter 9.

Outside the workplace, a number of technical steps toward making cities more liveable can be taken without waiting for further research or social reform. Comprehensive national firearms legislation as one means of controlling rising homicide rates is a case in point. The facts to support such legislation are clear and unequivocal and have been assembled, analyzed, and published as part of the Eisenhower Commission Report.[70] This evidence on the national level has been reinforced by studies of individual cities.[54] Gun control will obviously not eliminate social stress or interpersonal violence, but it can cope with the recent frightening increase in homicides, which has paralleled an increase in the manufacture and importation of guns. The fact that gun control faces strong opposition should be no cause for discouragement, since earlier campaigns for the abolition of child labor and the reduction of industrial hazards successfully overcame even stronger resistance on the part of industry.

There are other technological remedies at hand. The construction of safer automobiles, more rigorous application of long-established safety standards in industry, and the use of current scientific knowledge to define new standards are examples. Many of the frustrating delays of bureaucracy at all levels, from the post office to the penitentiary to the Supreme Court, could be reduced or eliminated by computerization. Systems analysis and other modern management techniques, applied to urban government, police, and courts, could increase efficiency and responsiveness.

One clear way to reduce risks to life in American cities would be to provide adequate pre- and postnatal care to all mothers and infants, particularly those who are exposed to increased risk because of medical or social factors. The New York study referred to above demonstrates conclusively that adequacy of care is strongly and consistently associated with reduction of prematurity and with survival of the infant, and that this relationship exists within comparable ethnic, educational, and risk groups.[78] There can be no doubt that extending services of this kind would save lives. In subsequent chapters, we shall consider some of the economic and organizational possibilities for bringing about more equitable access to health services.

But no amount of applied science will eliminate the urban ghetto and its train of human suffering. A large-scale technological experiment has actually been tried and proved a large-scale failure. "Urban renewal" was based on the naive premise that the elimination of deteriorated housing would remove slums and all that went with them. After a wasteful and sometimes tragic two decades, it is evident that slum clearance simply shifts poor people to non-slum areas, people who take their poverty and their stunted lives with them to create new slums, while their former homes are replaced by bleak office, bank, and civic buildings.[79]

Social action

True urban renewal must be based on our traditional commitment to democracy and social justice. Better housing must be planned as a means to a better life, not merely as a remedy for urban "blight." The police, the courts, and the prisons must be revitalized as agents of justice and social support rather than of punishment and ostracism. We can no longer afford to skimp on health and welfare services as an unwanted social burden but must instead willingly make them available as ways of liberating human lives.

Social reforms of the past were able to blunt the edge of urban poverty when it was a transient stage through which the immigrant passed. Jane Addams transplanted the British idea of a social "settlement house" to Chicago when she opened Hull House in 1889. Out of this center and others, such as Lillian Wald's Henry Street Settlement in New York City, came successful movements for juvenile courts, mothers' pensions, workmen's compensation and child labor laws. But today the settlement house seems a weak defense against riots in Watts and heroin pushing in Harlem.

The "War on Poverty," initiated during the Johnson administration, was a vigorous and imaginative effort to attack simultaneously several institutional sources of poverty from a headquarters in Washington. The poor were to be helped to overcome their own limitations. Education was to be enriched early for ghetto children, comprehensive health care centers established in the central cities and poor rural areas, family planning, vocational training, and legal services were to be offered, and the poor were to be enlisted in the making of decisions about their own future. Such an ambitious program was likely to fail, especially when administrations changed. Too much was attempted too soon, planning was too hurried, and waste, graft, inefficiency, and poor coordination took their toll. Predictable resistance came from local governments that had been excluded from the planning and the flow of federal money. Above all, the plan dealt with almost every aspect of poverty except the basic economic one. The reports are not all in, but at this time the best that can be said is that there were many failures and a few qualified successes.[80, 81, 82] Important lessons have been learned, and those lessons most relevant to health will be considered in more detail in Chapter 8.

Poverty has not yielded to the elimination of poor housing, nor to efforts to improve access to educational, health, legal, and other services. Having failed to abolish poverty by various indirect means, we are at last brought face to face with the painful fact that poverty is caused by a lack of money. More precisely, since wealth is the effective control of resources, including goods, services, and capital, poverty is the lack of control over such resources. As the gross national product is again growing, the persistence of extreme poverty in the United States becomes increasingly more shameful and politically intolerable.

The pattern of life in our urban slums, which at present alarms many citizens and can destroy those individuals who are forced to share it, will ultimately be humanized only by solving the economic riddle. Henry George stated the problem in 1880: "The association of poverty with progress is the great enigma of our times."[83] After an unprecedented period of economic expansion since World War II, extreme poverty continues to dog our footsteps, and the wealthiest one-fifth of the population continue to receive seven times as much income as the bottom one-fifth, just as they did 50 years ago.[84] The poor will probably not achieve a full measure of health until they can control a more equitable share of the resources. A broadening recognition of this imperative may be seen in the fact that some otherwise conservative politicians favor a form of negative income tax.

Because of the intimate relationship between urban health and the social and economic system of the country, we will return to the question of political action in the last chapter.

DERELICT PEOPLE

4

Some are born poor, some achieve poverty, and some have poverty thrust upon them. The preceding chapter dealt with the constricted lives of those who are born into the self-perpetuating cycle of urban poverty and cannot break out of it. Caught in the same dangerous social network are those smaller numbers of persons who reach poverty from middle-class beginnings as a result of deviant behavior, such as alcoholism, drug addiction, or compulsive gambling. But most individuals who become poor find the condition thrust upon them by the relentless progression of age or chronic illness, and aggravated by inflation and recession. For these people, as well as for those who enter the cycle at birth, ill health and poverty become reciprocal cause and effect.

HUMAN FRAILTY: AGE AND CHRONIC ILLNESS

Modern industrial cities are hard on the human constitution, and they offer cold comfort to citizens who become old, lame, and sick.

Miss Ada Holmes was born in 1875 in a small town near Cleveland, in which her father operated a hardware store. After high school, she considered going on to college, but this was difficult for a girl in 1893, and she settled for a secretarial school. She went to work as a secretary in the local bank and moved to the main office in 1910 when the bank merged with a larger one in Cleveland.

Over the years she became a trusted employee at the bank and subsequently in two or three secretarial jobs elsewhere. She remained a solitary person, however, living alone or with friends who enjoyed her company but found her a bit stubborn and quick-tempered. She never married.

She retired at 65, with some $10,000 in savings and her own comfortable old house. Her health seemed good, so she supplemented her savings by taking in as temporary boarders people who were attending the nearby Cleveland Clinic. Two years after retirement, however, she was belatedly discovered to have glaucoma. Two operations, when she was 69 and 72 years old, delayed the course of the disease, but soon after the second operation she lost all useful vision.

At this point she had no family left, other than cousins with whom she had lost touch, and she came to depend increasingly on a friend who lived with her. At age 77, now completely blind, she had a brief episode of confusion, which resulted in fractures of both wrists, and at the age of 80, she tripped one day as she was going out the door and broke her left hip. The fracture was pinned, and she was transferred to a rehabilitation hospital, where her convalescence was marked by periods of confusion and agitated behavior. A psychiatric consultant diagnosed chronic brain syndrome, characterized by memory loss and disorientation.

Her friend could no longer accept responsibility for her, and a guardianship was established with an attorney who arranged for her to be admitted to a proprietary nursing home with the ironic name of "Skyview Haven." This was a substantial old house in a deteriorating neighborhood, operated by a retired nurse who spent much of her time in Florida; it was inadequately staffed with practical nurses and aides. Miss Holmes's savings began to dwindle.

Because of her confusion, the busy staff kept her in bed most of the time or tied into a chair. She soon was unable to walk, and by the age of 83, she was incontinent and had to be fed. Fortunately, her earlier agitation decreased, and she was usually cheerful, though completely disoriented.

By the time she reached the age of 85, she had only funds sufficient for burial. The nursing home would not accept the minimal rates the state and federal Aid for Aged program paid (in 1961), so her guardian arranged for her admission to a state mental hospital. Her treatment there was little different from what it had been in the nursing home, but the shock of changing environments distressed her greatly. She died two weeks after being transferred.[1]

Legions of the aged

Miss Holmes's downward drift from middle-class self-sufficiency to poverty and death in a public institution is characteristic of the fate of a large and an increasing number of older persons in our modern urbanized world. One in ten Americans is now 65 years old or older, and 58 percent of these older persons are women. As in other developed countries, these proportions are higher than ever before. The present population structure is mainly the result of high fertility and the immigration of young people before 1900, with decreasing death rates since. Special prominence has been given to the current population of aged people by the succeeding lower fertility of the depression years. The proportion of persons over 65 will remain high until 1995 or 2000, with another large cohort reaching old age about 2015. For purposes of urban health planning, there is no reason to expect the numbers or proportion of old people to decrease for at least a generation.[2]

For many of the aged, chronic illness and disability determine the patterns of their lives, and the risk of developing most types of chronic illness increases rapidly with age. Of non-institutionalized people over 65, 86 percent report that they have one or more "chronic conditions." One-fifth say that they have limited mobility, and over one-third describe themselves as limited in a major activity, such as work or housekeeping. The leading causes of activity limitation among older persons are arthritis and rheumatism (21.2 percent), heart conditions (20.5 percent), and visual impairments (7.0 percent).[3,4]

The proportion of old people (65 years and over) is highest in non-metropolitan counties (11.4 percent), high in central city counties (10.8 percent), and distinctly lower in the suburbs (8.0 percent) (Table 4.1). The chronic conditions that limit activity among old people appear to be similar in metropolitan and non-metropolitan areas, though the complete picture is difficult to draw, since persons in nursing homes, chronic disease hospitals, and mental institutions have been studied separately from the National Health Survey, and their places of residence have not been reported.

Urban disability

We noted in the preceding chapter that the incidence of work injuries on the farm is higher than in the city and that this difference increases with age. A disability of movement seems likely to be a greater handicap to a farmer than to a bench or clerical worker. Heart disease and cancer, on the other hand, produce higher mortality rates in central city counties than elsewhere (Chapter 1). Death from both these diseases is usually preceded

Table 4.1
Percent distribution of persons by age and activity limitation status due to chronic conditions, United States (1969-1970)

	IN SMSA		*OUTSIDE SMSA*	
	Central City	*Suburban*	*Non-farm*	*Farm*
Percent of population aged 65 years and over[a]	10.8	8.0	11.4	10.5
Percent of population aged 65 years and over with no limitation of activity[b]	60.7	59.7	53.8	53.4
Percent of population aged 65 and over with limitation in amount or kind of major activity[b]	19.6	19.9	22.0	23.4

[a] U.S. Bureau of Census, United States Summary, 1970.
[b] National Center for Health Statistics, Vital and Health Statistics, Series 10, No. 80.

by months or years of increasingly incapacitating illness. Once recognized, these conditions can bar employment in the city at a stage when they might not prevent a farmer from working, because many employers will not hire an individual who may not be insurable and who may become incapacitated or be away from the job frequently. Old people in poor urban areas report rates of major chronic conditions that are markedly above the national average.[5] Since such conditions develop gradually, they tend to remove individuals from the labor market even before age forces retirement.

Thus, we can identify a significant rural population of old people unable to do farm work, often because of former injuries, and another, numerically larger population of urban old people, disabled by higher rates of such progressive illness as cancer and heart disease. These two groups of the aged are derelicts of the two great population trends of our recent history: the movement of young people away from farms and into the cities and the subsequent movement of successful young families from the inner city into the suburbs.

Social isolation

Old people, like racial minorities, are likely to become trapped in poor city neighborhoods. Some of the reasons are similar; these include job discrimination, mandatory retirement at age 62 or 65, lack or loss of skill, and lack of education, but some reasons are inherent in the aging process. The aged tend to stay on in the old neighborhood when it changes and thus become socially isolated. "Disengagement" has been identified by Cumming and Henry as an essentially normal process of withdrawal, which results in decreased interaction between the aging person and others in his social system.[6] As they point out, this process may be more psychologically healthy and mature than the alternative of a strained effort to continue youthful activities. But disengagement also has undeniably harmful social and economic consequences, since it diminishes material and human resources for the individual and converts a productive citizen into a dependent one.

Low family incomes in a large city are frequently associated with old age.[7, 8, 9] Loneliness and the pinch of poverty can be particularly acute in the urban environment. Costs of living are higher, and the urban aged are less likely to have the resource of living with relatives or in their own home than are comparable old people in non-metropolitan counties. Unmarried men over 65 in central cities, for example, have no relative present in the home in 70 percent of households, compared with 58 percent in non-metropolitan counties. In the cities, only 26 percent of these men own their homes, whereas outside of cities 44 percent do. Though the urban aged have higher incomes than average ($3,420 compared with $2,875 nationally for married couples in 1962), the difference is probably no advantage in terms of purchasing power, considering city rents alone.[10]

The social isolation of old people in modern American cities is greatly aggravated by inadequate and often deteriorating public transportation and housing. A study of the elderly poor in 13 communities in 1970 showed that transportation difficulties were a major problem, since "not only food, but health and medical care, church attendance, cultural activities, and recreation and social contacts depend upon adequate transportation facilities."[11] Looked at through the eyes of increasingly disabled older persons, a majority of whom are women, most urban transportation systems seem almost designed to immobilize them by means of such barriers as exposed, dangerous loading zones, high steps, erratic schedules, inconvenient routes, and rapidly increasing fares.

To own one's own home has been a life-long goal for many an American. But the achievement all too often turns sour. For the couple who have had children, their house is too big, with the family scattered. It ties up limited capital, and repairs become a heavy burden. Mortgage rates and property taxes rise steadily, eating up sporadic increases in Social Security income and entirely outdistancing fixed income from pensions and annuities. The "house-poor" owner, often a widow, finds it hard to sell a house in a deteriorating neighborhood, and the failure of urban renewal programs to provide adequate, low-rent public housing forces her to pay higher rents than she can afford. The savings of years are consumed by basic living expenses, and expenditure for private health care becomes one of the discretionary costs that can and therefore must be cut.

Institutionalization

A sizable proportion—3.7 percent—of Americans over 65 live in such institutions as hospitals, nursing homes, and residential homes.[12] For urban old people, a relative lack of human resources means that they are more likely than others to end their days in an institution. One reason for this difference is that disabled persons who live in metropolitan counties are less likely to receive home care than are those in non-metropolitan counties.[13] A survey of persons over 65 who were in institutions in western New York State found that old persons from urban areas were considerably more likely than old people elsewhere to be placed in a nursing home when their physical condition did not require it.[14] Similarly, it is estimated that 10 percent of nursing home residents in New York City are in nursing homes only because there are no appropriate social alternatives.[15]

But there are many more partially disabled old people who are not in institutions. A fire or a death occasionally brings to public attention an urban recluse—say an eccentric old man or a misanthropic old woman—who has been living for years as a hermit in the midst of a busy city. One study estimates that 7 to 10 percent of the urban population over 60 in the United States today need some form of continuing supervision and assistance from a community agency because they are more or less mentally incompetent and have no responsible relatives or friends. A search for such candidates for protective services in the city of Cleveland, using health and welfare agencies, housing authorities, and courts as sources of information, turned up 164 persons, most of whom proved to be over 75 years of age, female, white, native-born, and non-married (widowed, divorced, separated, or never married), with incomes rarely more than $150 and often less than $100 a month (in 1965).[16]

A survey of mental health of the residents of midtown Manhattan has confirmed the existence of an extensive urban population of isolated, aged, poor people, often mentally impaired, who have long been known to social workers, visiting nurses, and others who have had reasons to enter their homes. Age and poverty, the investigators found, are directly correlated with mental impairment, and the association, they believe, is brought about by the social processes of the poverty cycle.[17, 18]

Role-discontinuity is one such mechanism. The usual reasons for going out into the community no longer obtain as an old person relinquishes the roles of worker and parent. The raising of a family comes to an end, and work ceases. Interest in seeking new social or sexual partners wanes. The old person feels unwanted, and even the simple pleasures of shopping are curtailed by penury. Old people in cities often live alone or apart from their families, and chronic illness and disability may tie them down.

A second social process that aggravates the disability of the urban aged is their stigmatization as weak, dependent, and immobile—the opposite of the qualities of strength, self-reliance, and mobility so highly valued in American life. Such rules as early retirement have been introduced for the specific purpose of removing obstructive oldsters from the mainstream. The proportion of men over 65 who are gainfully employed has dropped from 70 percent in 1890 to 28 percent in 1968.[19] The combined effect of these age-associated changes, as Lerner and Anderson have observed, is that "during the middle and later years of life, the urbanized environment seems to be less conducive to health and longevity than is the rural environment."[20]

DOWN AND OUT: MENTAL ILLNESS

Does the stress of urban life actually bring out or produce mental illness? Plausible though this concept may be, it is difficult to document. Definitions are not uniform, and statistics from different sources cannot be compared. Death is rarely attributed directly to mental illness, so mortality rates are not useful. The National Health Survey excludes persons in institutions, with the result that the 600,000 patients in mental hospitals are not described in demographic terms comparable to the terms used for other illnesses and disabilities. Age, poverty, the downward social drift of the elderly, and possibly migration are all related to mental illness and must be taken into account in analyzing its relationship to urban residence.

Despite these difficulties, a few studies have been made of this subject, and most workers have reported that urban rates of mental illness exceed those of rural areas. A study of newly diagnosed psychotics in Texas for the years 1951 and 1952, for example, showed "urban" (over 2,500 population) rates to be twice as high as rural rates, after adjustment of the data of age, sex, and subculture.[21] First admissions to mental hospitals have been shown to occur consistently more frequently among urban residents, whether the diagnosis is cerebral arteriosclerosis and senility, psychosis, or other disorders. Another well documented and possibly related fact is that persons born in another country are more likely to be admitted to mental hospitals than are natives of the United States.[22] Since most immigrants first settled in seaboard cities, the vulnerability of the foreign-born and that of urban residents appear to be associated. Blacks had lower first-admission rates than whites in the early part of this century, particularly in the rural south, but as they have moved into northern cities, their hospitalization rates have come to equal those of whites.[23] A move into the city may be precipitated by social and psychological stress, and it also brings the urban in-migrant into contact with new kinds of stress. The in-migrant from rural areas is consistently reported to have a higher rate of mental illness than is found among settled urban residents.[24, 25]

Minority status as a foreigner, a black, or a person bred on a farm, combined with the stresses of moving into a strange city, may contribute to strange behavior commonly identified as mental illness.[26]

Some of the higher rates for urban mental hospitalization can be accounted for by the fact that mental hospitals are more accessible in the city. We will return to this question in the next chapter, but the higher urban rates cannot be entirely explained in this way. As with other aspects of poverty, mental illness can be found concentrated in certain segments of the non-hospitalized urban population. When metropolitan areas are compared with nonmetropolitan counties, the prevalence of disabling mental and nervous conditions and of symptoms of psychological distress seems to be similar or even slightly lower in the metropolitan areas.[27, 28] But when we examine the prevalence of serious mental illness among specific groups, it is clear that these conditions are relatively more frequent in the lower social classes, among non-whites, among the unemployed, among the aged, and among those individuals who are moving down the social scale.

A common psychological mechanism that could explain the tendency to mental illness in all these groups is the feeling of powerlessness that prevails among the poor.[26, 29] A poor person with a marginal social adjustment may be sustained, even in the absence of supporting family, by a few friendly neighbors, shop-keepers, or church members. But the physical growth of the city and the enlargement and depersonalization of its institutions and services constantly endanger the fragile structure of such a life. Repeated deprivations–the loss of a job, advancing age, deterioration of the neighborhood, and the movement of friends and associates to the suburbs–reduce the sense of control over one's destiny. Whether mental illness is considered a failure of adjustment on the part of the individual or a manifestation of social pathology, the contemporary inner city seems almost planned to foster and accentuate it.

SALVAGING PEOPLE

Chronic illness, senility, and mental illness lead to poverty and are aggravated in turn by the social isolation and impotence of poverty. What can be done for these millions of derelicts adrift in the backwaters of urban life? The humanitarian objectives can be simply stated: We must provide a decent life for individuals who are unable to support themselves because of age, disability, or illness.

What technical and scientific means can we command, and what social reforms are possible to achieve this goal?

Social engineering

Some of the engineering problems involved in getting derelict people back into the mainstream, though challenging, seem to be readily soluble once we have agreed upon the need for such services and are ready to bear the cost. Fast, safe, cheap urban transportation, for example, would immediately improve the lives of the elderly and the chronically disabled. Our present urban transportation system, with its heavy dependence on the automobile, is out of the reach of such people. Several imaginative proposals and experiments have been put forth. Linked rail and bus systems, with flexible routes and automated schedules, safer, more pleasant vehicles, and comfortable, protected waiting areas are technically feasible today.

Public transportation should be free, or nearly free, to the aged and the disabled.[30] Financing of urban transportation is clearly inadequate when confined to a local taxation or profit-making base.[31, 32] Federal revenues in the massive highway trust funds are an obvious source to tap, and Congress has moved in this direction, against strong resistance from powerful oil and automotive lobbies. The Urban Mass Transit Act of 1964, amended in 1966 and 1968, were important legislative steps in this direction, but present funds are grossly inadequate. The energy crisis, which was brought sharply into focus in 1973, makes the need for better public transportation clear and urgent.

The housing problem also offers opportunities for architectural and engineering creativity, though experience also dramatically shows how wrong a drawing-board "solution" can be if it does not take into account the ultimate human purpose of the structure. The boxlike, high-rise public housing building, exemplified at its worst by the Pruitt-Igoe Project in Saint Louis, has been literally attacked and nearly destroyed by the people assigned to live in it because it did not provide "defensible space"—a secure and dignified habitation for human beings.[33]

National goals for better housing were clearly enunciated in the Housing Act of 1949: "The realization as soon as feasible of the goal of a decent home and a suitable living environment for every American family." As we noted in the last chapter, however, the massive urban renewal program has failed to provide adequate low cost housing for the poor and the elderly. As many as 5.7 million Americans were still living in substandard housing in 1967.[34] Jane Jacobs called attention to the dehumanizing effect of modern cities and recent urban planning, and a new wave of architectural design acknowledged the need to restore the city to human dimensions.[35] Great obstacles remain, however. Space allocated to housing reduces the space available for industry and other revenue-producing uses. Those who live in new urban housing increase the demand for public services, which cost more than regressive property taxes can be made to yield. Obsolete building codes and union rules inhibit new construction methods and keep costs up.

In spite of these difficulties, as with those related to transportation, there are exciting possibilities a real national commitment could unlock. As soon as one begins to put human needs ahead of such commercial considerations as land-use, traffic flow, and cheap construction, the appropriate dimensions begin to emerge. Homes for old people in the city should be small, functionally designed living units, private and protected from traffic and crime but linked to transportation and arranged in socially meaningful neighborhoods with convenient recreation, shopping, and other services.[36] Urban old people wish to live in contact with the world, not segregated in rural "homes" or boxed up in high-rise apartments. At the same time, the residents need to be able to call for help when they need it and to have readily available services, such as nursing and medical care, which they need more than young people do. The design of public housing along these lines has barely been started in this country. Planning, financing, and supporting adequate housing for the poor and the elderly will require responsible action at federal, state and local levels.[37] Massachusetts has accepted this responsibility more fully than most other states, and the developing outlines of the necessary public policy can be seen there.[34]

Those individuals who are old and disabled but still able to exist independently will live more decent lives if they can have better homes and better transportation. But there will still be many who need more or complete care. Health care resources are the subject of the next chapter, but here we must acknowledge the urgent need for reform of those services that most people who become physically disabled or mentally ill will ultimately depend upon: the nursing homes and mental hospitals that house more than a million people. With too few exceptions, these are among our most disgraceful institutions. The tales of overcrowding, inadequate staffing, brutalizing institutional practices, and plain neglect are so familiar that we become inured to them.[38] Can these institutions be humanized, along with transportation and housing? Again, there are definite advantages to be gained by better design. But the doors of the state mental hospital cannot really be unlocked nor the shabby firetrap of a nursing home replaced by a respectable place in which to live until we tackle more broadly based social reform.

In the early 1960's, before Medicare, there were estimated to be over half a million persons in nursing and personal care homes. Two-thirds of them were over 75 years old; roughly one-fifth were confined to bed and another one-fifth limited to a single room.[39] Ownership of these homes was mainly in private hands, with 90 percent of the homes and 70 percent of the beds classified as proprietary. Two-thirds of the proprietary homes had no one more highly trained than a licensed practical nurse on the staff, and 40 percent of the patients had not seen a physician for over a month. The situation was described as "a medical care vacuum."[40]

The Medicare law (1965) provided funds for post-hospital care and established minimum standards for "extended care facilities" and "home health agencies" to meet in order to qualify for payment. The prospect of public funds led to the construction of many new nursing homes, some of which have already failed. Those homes that have met the new criteria and managed to survive have had a favorable influence on the quality of nursing home care. Surveys of nursing homes in Massachusetts in 1965 and 1969 showed that there had been much more compliance with state standards and that the homes had improved in terms of staffing, plant, services, and records, but not, unfortunately, in respect to the personal care of the patients as judged by their appearance.[41]

The need for an entirely new approach to the delivery of community mental services has been recognized, growing out of experimentation with "open hospitals" and "therapeutic communities" after World War II.[42] President Kennedy's personal interest in mental retardation led to Congressional authorization of federal matching funds for the construction of community mental health and mental retardation facilities in 1963. A guiding principle has become to "shift the arena from the remote state hospital system of long-term institutional care to comprehensive services within the local community." The new concept of a mental health "center" is a coordinated set of services, ranging from screening and counseling to intensive hospital treatment, aimed at keeping the patient functioning in the community and avoiding custodial care.[43]

The numbers of patients in state and county mental hospitals have been reduced by 40 percent and admissions by nearly 50 percent over the decade of the 1960's, though there is no good evidence that nursing home, home care, and ambulatory services have been expanded enough to provide for those who have been discharged. Prolonged treatment of any sort for mental illness is specifically excluded from coverage by Medicare and by private insurers. The public responsibility for long-term psychiatric care has traditionally been lodged with the state, and this unwelcome responsibility is frequently discharged at minimum cost. Most state mental hospitals are staffed by physicians who were trained in foreign medical schools. Salaries remain low, staff positions are often unfilled, and only the geographic isolation of many of these large institutions keeps what are often deplorable conditions from the public view. The President of the American Psychiatric Association, acknowledging the continued existence of serious deficiencies in mental health services, has called for the creation of a new Joint Commission on Mental Illness and Health to reassess the problem on a national basis.[44]

Something to live on

Old people in American cities continue to list income as their leading problem, in spite of the fact, surprising to many, that the United States has one of the most extensive and firmly established systems of compulsory social insurance in the world. The Social Security Program (Old-Age, Survivors, and Disability Insurance) is a system of earnings replacement and income maintenance, which arose out of the stringent need of the Depression. In the face of widespread unemployment, Congress was compelled to recognize that the interaction of poverty and old age meant literal starvation for many citizens. Private enterprise was paralyzed, and the only hope for survival of the unemployable lay in government action. The law was enacted in 1935, despite many misgivings, and the first payments were made in 1940.

Still widely considered to be an insurance program, Social Security is in fact a system of transfer payments, in which money collected from the current working population by an employer-employee payroll tax is used to pay benefits to others who have retired or who cannot work because of dependency status or disability. Social Security funds are held in trust and administered by a bureau, which is ponderous but, on the whole, remarkably efficient and fair. Over a 27-year period, the Social Security Administration distributed $180 billion in benefits without a single serious incident of fraud or deception.[45] The political acceptability of Social Security is demonstrated by the fact that, despite conservative objections, no administration in the last 40 years has attempted to repeal or even to restrict the program. On the contrary, payments and coverage have been periodically extended under both Republican and Democratic administrations. Perhaps the most significant testimony to the durability of the program is the fact that when the first major step was taken toward a national health insurance program–the Medicare law of 1965–it was written as an amendment to the Social Security Act.

At present, Social Security provides fixed monthly payments to the aged, to surviving spouses, and to those with total disability. Of individuals over 65, 79 percent were receiving benefits in 1970, and the proportion will rise to 84 percent in 1980.[46] Persons not covered may receive public assistance (state and federal matching funds), which varies greatly from one state to another, or they may live on government or private pensions.

The Social Security program has two objectives: income maintenance for retired or disabled wage-earners and the elimination of poverty for those individuals who have never been able to support themselves. The payroll tax is an accepted mechanism for meeting the first objective. When the program is amended, however, as it has been, to provide benefits for all those past 72 and those who have worked only for brief periods or at very low wages, it is clear that the second objective would be more appropriately met from general revenues than from a payroll tax. As it now operates, the payroll withholding tax is regressive, since fixed upper limits of contribution mean that low-income workers contribute a higher proportion of their earnings. Thus, a tax system that was devised to assist the elderly poor actually penalizes these same persons during their working years. Extension of the Social Security program, therefore, if it continues to occur as it has for 35 years, will be on a more equitable tax base if it evolves toward direct support of all dependent persons out of general revenues.[47]

Social Security has unquestionably blunted the impact of poverty on the elderly citizens of this nation, but it has certainly not eliminated that poverty. Fixed allowances, inadequate to begin with, fall further behind as inflation continues. Testimony in Congressional hearings in 1969 showed that the average Social Security benefits of a couple retiring in 1950 met one-half their estimated cost of living then, but only one-third in 1967.[48] A 20 percent increase in 1972 did little more than compensate for increased costs due to inflation.

The working out of a satisfactory income maintenance program for the increasing numbers of elderly people in this country is part of the larger national task of extending social reform. Special aspects of the problem of the elderly that will have to be taken into account include the role of private pensions, the need to move beyond the insurance concept, choices between income maintenance and specific benefits, and the conflict between personal need for continued meaningful work and economic pressures toward earlier retirement. One reason Social Security has been so well accepted is that it is free of the degrading means test associated with public assistance. The idea of a negative income tax has been proposed as a fair and dignified means of assuring a minimum income to everyone.[49, 50, 51]

Medicare

The passage of Medicare in 1965 established for the first time in this country a compulsory health insurance program on a national basis, funded, for the most part, like Social Security, and covering virtually all of the elderly population. Though the step was taken with great caution, it was widely recognized as a major though partial victory in a 50-year battle for national health insurance. The impact of the law has already been great. Virtually all the elderly population is covered for hospitalization, and 96 percent of eligible individuals have also accepted the "voluntary" supplemental benefit insurance program (Part B), which provides limited coverage for physicians' fees, extended care (nursing home), home care, and other services. The insurance industry eventually supported Medicare, since it had learned that it could not market health insurance at premium rates adequate to meet the increasing needs of older people. Hospitals welcomed the law as a reliable source of payment for the aged, who fill a disproportionate number of beds, though they recognize that along with government money come new requirements for cost accounting, utilization review, and other types of unfamiliar and unwelcome external regulation.[52] A major drawback of Medicare health reimbursement, from the point of view of the elderly and disabled, is the petty bureaucratic system of coinsurance, deductibles, and assignment of payment intended, with no supporting evidence of effectiveness, to discourage "unnecessary" use of health services. The over-all impact of Medicare and its controversial companion law, Medicaid (Title XIX)[53] cannot yet be assessed, but an indication of its importance is the fact that in the first year after the law was passed, the Federal share of national health expenditures rose from 25 to 35 percent.[54]

Complex though financing living expenses and health services for the elderly may be, it is only part of what must be done to provide for individuals who are now isolated and poor in our cities and to prevent others from succeeding them. The Older Americans Act of 1965, with subsequent revisions, has enunciated such problems as nutrition, the idleness of retirement, and the need for geriatric research, but the measures adopted have been on too small a scale to be effective.[55] True urban renewal has not been achieved. The nursing home "industry" has profited from government funding, and formal standards are beginning to be enforced in some states (Massachusetts), but the beds that are needed are not available, the costs are prohibitive for many, and most homes remain impersonal institutions. Home care services, almost non-existent before Medicare, have been given an important stimulus but still lag far behind what is provided in Great Britain and Scandinavia. Many patients have been discharged from state mental hospitals, but we do not know where they have gone or how they are faring.

Thus, the citizens of the United States, through their Congress, have accepted part of the responsibility for salvaging the lives of the aged and other economically dependent persons, though the terms of the social contract are too often arbitrary, restrictive, and demeaning. An adequate income, safe, decent homes, skilled help in time of need–these seem reasonable and feasible goals. Close to our grasp, they continue to elude us. A good beginning was made in 1935, and another step occurred in 1965, but the work is not complete.

The family

Though the development of industrial cities has tended in many ways to increase the social isolation of the elderly, there have also been compensatory social changes, which may open the way to healthier living patterns. A recent study of old people in three industrialized societies shows that, because of increasing survival at all ages plus a trend toward earlier marriage, 44 percent of Americans over 65 belong to a three-generation family, and 32 percent are part of four living generations. Only 3 percent of older people have no child, spouse, or sibling alive.[56] American families, compared to those in Britain and Denmark, tend more to help maintain separate households for older couples, and older people in this country seem to value and strive to maintain independence and physical mobility later in life.[57]

The family, therefore, constitutes an important resource for a large majority of older Americans, and family members, even when they are not present in the same household, can provide social and psychological reinforcement, which may be more important than financial support.[58] Inner resources and a positive self-image developed during a lifetime of family association can be sustained by a small but essential amount of contact.

The marked predominance of women among the aged has led to the interesting proposal that unattached older women could elect to become part of an "affiliated family." Such an arrangement would increase the older person's human resources, enable her to regain social significance in the role of a grandmother, and permit the younger mother more time for continued education and a career. Other types of affiliated relationship are also possible, all with the essential feature of mutual support and maintenance of the older person in a healthy, non-institutional setting.[59]

The family, as the primordial social group, probably serves a more important function in sustaining older and disabled people than is generally recognized nowadays. Living alone does not necessarily mean being alone. Even in the city, personal and telephone visits with children and siblings can form vital links with life and reality.

The modern American family is tending to become vertically rather than horizontally extended. Though divorce rates are rising, so are marriage rates, and the married state is still decidedly the norm.[60] The family of the future will probably be more scattered and complex, but in one sense it may be stronger than it was in the past, since entering and leaving will be more a matter of choice. As increased voluntary control over the reproductive functions of the family offer the potential of healthier children, so increased flexibility in relationships with older persons could extend the socialization function of the family to include the reintegration of the elderly along with the growth and development of younger members.

GETTING CARE 5

The same urban qualities that maximize the exchange of goods and money also facilitate the interaction between health care providers and consumers. It takes capital to build a major hospital, and such a hospital needs a large and conveniently located population to keep its beds filled. The complicated mix of talents and training required to staff a modern medical center can be found in a city, but not in a small town. People exposed to the stress and clash of urban life have a need for round-the-clock emergency services, and the social energy of their life provides the means to operate these services.

But the urban health care system is full of inequities. Complex feats, such as X-ray visualization of the coronary arteries, are performed with skill and technical perfection, whereas ordinary tasks, such as making sure that all school children are adequately immunized, are often neglected and mismanaged. Poor people living in the shadow of many world-famous hospitals cannot afford to use their services.

Most of these paradoxes, which range from inconvenience to

great social injustice, result from difficulties in gaining access to health services. In a large city, barriers to the use of services are sometimes geographic, more often economic, and occasionally related to other social differences, such as race. Like other technological functions, the delivery of health care has developed unevenly, strongly influenced by the needs and convenience of the providers and very little by those of the consumer. In this chapter we will consider some of the reasons why different citizens have such widely differing access to the health care system. In the next chapter, we will take up the more difficult question of the effectiveness of services: Is the city dweller who obtains access healthier than others who do not, and, if so, is the difference related to the service?

THE AVAILABLE RESOURCES

Services that are closer are generally more accessible. In an early American epidemiological study (1852), Jarvis observed that admission rates to mental hospitals vary inversely with the distance between the patient's residence and the institution.[1] "Jarvis' Law" has recently been reconfirmed for first admissions to state mental hospitals in Connecticut, and this study has also shown that the effect of proximity can be demonstrated at all ages and that it is independent of race, severity of illness, and financial status.[2] Admissions to general hospitals have also been shown to obey this rule.[3, 4]

Though simple distance evidently influences the use of hospitals, travel time may be more important in the use of ambulatory services. A recent study, which takes both factors into account, demonstrates that for those who live close to the central business district the average time required to reach the dentist or the physician is greater than it is for those who live elsewhere. Part of this difference can be attributed to the fact that public transportation in many American cities is slower than the private automobile.[5]

Hospital services, physicians, nurses, dentists, and other health workers tend to be where patients, supporting services, and educational facilities are available. The ratio of physicians to the population of the United States was estimated as 166 per 100,000 in 1970. This ratio began to rise slowly in 1950 and has accelerated since 1965. The proportion of physicians in private practice was declining until 1967.[6] At that time the classification of type of practice was changed, and there was no significant change in the proportion of physicians "rendering patient care" from 1968 through 1972.[7] But these physicians are not evenly distributed. The ratio of physicians to population in metropolitan counties is twice what it is in the rest of the nation (Table 5.1). The only physicians who are evenly distributed are general practitioners, and their numbers were rapidly declining until the recent renaissance of family medicine. Studies of individual cities, such as Boston,[8] Cleveland,[9] and Chicago,[10] show that within a metropolitan county the distribution of physicians also varies widely. Physi-

Table 5.1
Percent distribution of non-federal physicians and population, United States (1972)

	Metropolitan Counties	*Non-metropolitan Counties*
POPULATION (207,486,300)	73.6	26.4
Total physicians (325,789)[a]	86.1	13.9
Patient care physicians (269,095)	85.5	14.5
Office-based practice:		
General practice (49,265)	67.4	32.6
Specialty practice (149,709)	87.8	12.2
Hospital based practice (70,121)	93.4	6.6
Other professional activity (24,228)[a]	93.2	6.8
Inactive (20,110)	81.3	18.7
Not classified (12,365)	93.2	6.8

Source: G. A. Roback, *Distribution of Physicians in the United States, 1972,* Vol. 2/Metropolitan Areas (Chicago: American Medical Association, 1973), Table A.

[a] Includes medical teaching, administration, research, and other.

cians are leaving the poorer sections of the central cities, except where they are clustered around a large medical center, and moving to the suburbs with their prosperous middle-class patients. In some areas of large cities, populations of 100,000 or more have ratios of physicians to population lower than any reported from the east south central states, where the lowest regional and state concentrations of physicians in the United States are found.[10, 11]

The national supply of dentists dropped slightly from 49.9 active dentists per 100,000 population in 1950 to 46.5 in 1968. Metropolitan counties generally have dentist to population ratios 50 percent or more higher than non-metropolitan counties. The ratio in the New York City metropolitan area was 82.5 in 1970, whereas that in non-metropolitan Mississippi was 21.4.[12] The average length of waiting time for a dental appointment is reported to be shorter the larger the city.

Nurses are also very unevenly distributed.[13] New Hampshire had 474 nurses per 100,000 population in 1966, whereas Arkansas had only 119. Greater metropolitan areas averaged 328, but isolated rural counties only 126.[14]

Hospital facilities, at first glance, seem to be better distributed than physicians, since the general hospital bed to population ratios in the two types of counties are similar (Table 5.2). Closer examination of the figures, however, shows that the average size of metropolitan hospitals is three times greater, and that the average non-metropolitan hospital contains only 76 beds, which is below the size (approximately 100 beds) that can be efficiently operated and still provide the essential services of a general hospital.[15] Even metropolitan hospitals average only twice this minimal size (226 beds). When one thinks of the many, very large central city hospitals, it is evident that a majority of hospitals in the United States are small and inadequate or inefficient and that such hospitals are very often the only ones readily available to persons who live away from large cities. Conversely, large hospitals with the highly specialized facilities and services often identified with high quality care are located, with very few exceptions, in large urban areas. The apparent similarity between metropolitan and non-metropolitan counties in terms of hospital bed to population ratio does not mean that metropolitan and non-metropolitan resi-

Table 5.2
Distribution of hospitals, hospital beds, and population, United States (1972)

	Metropolitan Counties	Non-metropolitan Counties
Population (207,486,300), percent	73.6	26.4
Number of hospitals (5,895),[a] percent	49.1	50.9
Number of hospital beds (883,192),[a] percent	74.0	26.0
Average number of beds per hospital	226	76
Average number of beds per 1,000 population	4.28	4.19

Source: G. A. Roback, *Distribution of Physicians in the United States, 1972,* Vol. 2/Metropolitan Areas (Chicago: American Medical Association, 1973), Table A.

[a] Excludes federal, long-term, psychiatric, tuberculosis, chronic disease and/or convalescent, and children's hospitals; and hospital departments of an institution.

dents have comparable access to the full range of hospital services. Potentially, at least, this access is better for the urban resident.

USE OF SERVICES

If proximity alone determined use, the fact that health services are relatively concentrated in urban areas would lead us to expect higher rates of use in those areas. For visits to physicians and dentists, this prediction is generally borne out. For hospital admissions and length of stay, however, the effect of proximity is distorted by other factors. The use of services in different residential areas is clearly affected by the personal characteristics of the population served, such as age and sex, which imply different kinds and severity of illness. Other important factors imply social differences in the ability or the means required to make use of available services. Income and education are factors of this sort, and race, when it is the basis for segregation or discrimination, is another factor.[16] In order to understand the patterns of use of health services in urban areas, it will be necessary to consider the interplay of all these elements. The National Health Survey is beginning to provide data that permit a first look at this problem, though the sporadic way in which the data are published limits analysis. The interaction of all these factors (and others), which ultimately determine whether an individual will visit a particular doctor or be admitted to a particular hospital on a given day, can be described only in outline, but that description is revealing.

Ambulatory care

Persons who live in metropolitan areas visit a physician or a dentist more often than those who live elsewhere (Table 5.3). This pattern of average urban-related use is consistent for physician visits at all ages, and for families of all sizes, which constitute 95 percent of the population. Physician visits, as one would expect, are more frequent than average for the newborn and for women of childbearing age, and they increase for both sexes with advancing age.

Physician and dental visits, which are rarely covered by health insurance, might also be expected to vary with income. This is the case for dental visits at all ages[17] and for physician visits below the age of 14.[18] For the general population, however, the highest rates of physician visits are found, surprisingly enough, among the poorest segments (those with family incomes under $5,000 in 1969), the lowest among those with marginal incomes ($5,000 to $6,999) and intermediate rates among those with middle and upper incomes ($7,000 and over).[19] Income may generally be considered an index of social class, suggesting differences in background and health-care habits as well as available resources. Education of the head of household, another class index, is directly related to frequency of physician visits in the pediatric age range and tends to parallel income relationships generally.[20]

A recent study of nine urban poverty areas, using the same survey questions as those used in the National Health Survey, offers a rare opportunity to compare use of services by the poor in the inner city with their use elsewhere.[21] Compared to poor people in

Table 5.3
Use of physician and dental services, United States (1969-1970; 1963)[a]

	IN SMSA[a]		*OUTSIDE SMSA*[a]	
	Central city	*Outside central city*	*Non-farm*	*Farm*
Physician visits (per person per year, age-adjusted)[b]	4.7 (± 0.08)	4.6 (± 0.06)	4.2 (± 0.07)	3.1 (± 0.16)
Persons with one or more physician visits in a year (percent, unadjusted)[b]	70.6 (± 0.3)	72.8 (± 0.3)	69.4 (± 0.3)	62.4 (± 0.7)
Dental visits (per person per year, age-adjusted)[b]	1.6 (± 0.04)	1.8 (± 0.04)	1.2 (± 0.04)	1.1 (± 0.09)
Persons with one or more dental visits in a year (percent, unadjusted)[b]	44.1 (± 0.3)	51.5 (± 0.3)	41.6 (± 0.3)	41.5 (± 0.7)
First medical visit during pregnancy in first trimester (percent)[c]	36.7 (± 0.3)		32.1 (± 0.4)	

[a] Values within parentheses are standard errors.
[b] National Center for Health Statistics, Vital and Health Statistics, DHEW Publication No. (HRA) 74-1513, Series 10, No. 86 (data from 1969-70).
[c] National Center for Health Statistics, Vital and Health Statistics, PHS Publication No. 1000, Series 22, No. 4 (data from 1963).

the country as a whole, the poor in urban areas, particularly those with chronic conditions, were found to be high users of physician services. Residents of these areas who did not report chronic conditions, on the other hand, had below average rates of physician visits. These discrepancies suggest that the inner city poor make relatively few routine or health maintenance visits, particularly for their children, since, where the poor live, doctors are hard to find, and costs are high. When illness does occur, however, it may be more severe because of neglect and therefore require more frequent physician visits. Another possible explanation of the relatively high rates among the poor is that fragmentation and inefficiency of services necessitate more visits to deal with one person's sometimes multiple problems.

An important question about which we lack information is what proportion of ambulatory care is furnished by private practitioners, organized groups, and hospital clinics and emergency rooms in urban, suburban, and non-metropolitan areas. A threefold increase in the use of hospital outpatient departments has occurred in the 50 largest cities of the United States over the past 20 years, and a fivefold increase in the use of emergency rooms.[22] This trend has been detected even within a prepaid group practice in Portland, Oregon, where the ratio of appointment to walk-in visits increased 26 percent in 7 years.[23]

Outpatient clinics are more commonly used as a source of ambulatory care in large cities than elsewhere in the country, but the increasing use of emergency rooms as a substitute for clinics or the doctor's office seems to be more prevalent outside the large cities (Table 5.4).

Factors contributing to the trend toward more use of clinics and emergency rooms have been the out-migration of private physicians from the inner city to the suburbs, insurance that covers "emergency" but not routine visits, an increasing need or desire on the part of physicians for X-ray and laboratory services, which are most readily available in hospitals, and geographic and temporal convenience. The increased service load this trend places on hospitals has been particularly difficult to handle, since ambulatory care is infrequently covered by patient insurance and unevenly and inadequately covered by public funds. The resulting pressures give the impression that hospitals provide most of the ambulatory service to city populations. This is probably not the case, since less than 10 percent of physician visits nationally take place in hospital clinics or emergency rooms,[17] and recorded visits to the hospitals of one large city amount to less than 10 percent of the estimated physician visits in that city. Studies of the use of ambulatory health services by different types of urban residents

Table 5.4
Ambulatory care in hospitals of the 50 largest cities of the United States (1969)

	Fifty largest cities	*United States*
Population, percent	20	100
Hospital beds, percent	40	100
Outpatient visits per 1,000 population per year	1,138	571
Outpatient visits per inpatient admission	6.1	4.2
Emergency room visits as percent of total visits	27.4	34.0

Source: N. Piore and D. Lewis, "Patterns of hospital outpatient use in fifty cities of the United States" (Paper presented to American Public Health Association, Atlantic City, N.J., November 16, 1972).

indicate that these patterns are quite complex. More than one-half the patients attending one outpatient department, for example, also had a private physician.[24]

Racial differences in the use of physician services are probably independent of income and education. White persons consistently make more visits to physicians than non-whites, even in comparable income groups. Thus, the average number of physician visits per person per year for those families with incomes below $5,000 (1966-1967) was 4.7 for whites and 3.1 for non-whites. Above this income level, the comparable figures are 4.5 for whites and 3.1 for non-whites. The study of inner city poverty areas referred to above showed regional differences in the use of physicians by the urban poor, with the lowest rates in the South. This may reflect lack of available physicians, lingering racial discrimination, or other local conditions.

Hospitalization

The use of hospitals is less clearly related to urban residence than is the use of physicians. Briefly, those who live outside metropolitan areas but not on farms (i.e., in towns and small cities) have the highest rates of discharge from short-stay hospitals. Farm residents have the lowest discharge rates, and metropolitan residents are intermediate in terms of both discharge rates and length of stay (Table 5.5).

These patterns result from the interplay of many factors, including the personal and social characteristics of patients, that were considered relative to physician and dental visits. Discharge rates and length of stay both increase with age, and discharge rates (with relatively short stays) increase during the childbearing years for women. Age adjustment of the data, however, does not change the observed residential differences.

Race has a paradoxical effect. Whites have almost 20 percent higher discharge rates but more than 20 percent shorter average stays.[25] It appears that it is more difficult for non-whites to be admitted to the hospital but that they stay longer once admitted, whether because of delay in treatment, lack of adequate home care, or because only the most seriously ill are admitted. Differences in the quality of hospital services available to whites and non-whites may also influence these measures of use.

The cost of hospitalization is the largest item in the health care budget. Paradoxically, poor people (under $4,000 family income) have significantly more hospital admissions and longer stays than do people with higher incomes. These differences may

Table 5.5
Rates of discharge and length of stay in short-stay hospitals by area of residence, United States (1968-1969)

	IN SMSA[a]	*OUTSIDE SMSA*[a]	
		Non-farm	*Farm*
Rate of discharge (per 1,000 persons per year)	120.8 (± 0.8)	138.6 (± 2.8)	108.8 (± 6.2)
Average length of stay (days)	9.5 (± 0.1)	8.4 (± 0.2)	9.8 (± 0.6)

Source: National Center for Health Statistics, Vital and Health Statistics, DHEW Publication No. (HSM) 72-1026, Series 10, No. 70, 1972.

[a] Values within parentheses are standard errors.

be observed at all ages except over age 65, when Social Security and, now, Medicare, have some equalizing effect. Here, as with physician visits, income may be significant as an index of social status and related health care needs as well as a measure of buying power. It appears that the very poor and the well-to-do have comparatively good access to hospital services, whereas those with marginal incomes, who can neither qualify for public assistance nor afford insurance, direct payment, or time away from work, tend to avoid or curtail hospitalization whenever they can.

Approximately 80 percent of the civilian, non-institutional population of the United States under the age of 65 had some form of insurance that would pay for some hospitalization in 1968, and this figure had increased from 67 percent in 1959.[26] Insurance coverage increases with urbanization. In metropolitan counties, 81.3 percent of those under 65 have partial or complete hospital coverage, whereas outside these counties the comparable figures are 74.4 percent in non-farm communities and 61.9 percent on farms. This pattern arises from the fact that most hospital insurance is purchased through unions or big companies, which are concentrated in large cities. The likelihood of having hospital and surgical insurance increases directly with family income, most markedly at the lower income levels, and it increases also with the education of the head of the family. Almost 50 percent more whites than non-whites hold such insurance.

For people over the age of 65, Medicare provides hospital coverage and some ambulatory and home care benefits for almost the entire population. Evidence of the relationship between available financing and the use of hospitals appeared following the introduction of Medicare in 1965. Both hospital discharges and length of stay jumped by one-quarter for the elderly population (Table 5.6). This increase cannot be entirely attributed to the new coverage, however, since there had also been a 28 percent increase in discharge rate for this population group in the preceding 5-year period (1959-1964).

Medicare did, however, have a striking effect on the use of hospitals by those who live on farms. Farm residents had clearly experienced the lowest rates of discharge and the shortest hospital stays before the new law, whereas after its passage their use of

Table 5.6
Hospital discharge rates and average length of stay for persons 65 years and over, by area of residence, before and after Medicare, United States (1963-1969)

	SMSA	*OUTSIDE SMSA*	
		Non-farm	*Farm*
Discharge rate, 1963-1965 (per 1,000 persons)	165.2	209.1	176.0
Discharge rate, 1968-1969 (per 1,000 persons)	209.1	267.6	277.3
percent change	+ 26.6	+ 19.1	+ 57.6
Average length of stay, 1963-1965 (days)	13.8	11.7	9.0
Average length of stay, 1968-1969 (days)	17.0	13.4	13.1
percent change	+23.2	+ 14.5	+ 45.6

Source: National Center for Health Statistics, Vital and Health Statistics, DHEW Publication No. (HSM) 72-1026, Series 10, No. 70, 1972, Table G.

hospitals equaled or slightly exceeded that of persons in towns and small cities. Since we know that farm residents as a group are the least likely to have health insurance, it is probable that the very large increase in their use of hospitals following Medicare represented a need for services, not manifested earlier because the elderly farm population could not afford elective hospitalization.[27] This experience indicates that some of the recent increase in hospital use is the result of cleaning up a backlog of unmet need. Is some of the increase also the consequence of using funded (and expensive) hospital care instead of less adequately funded ambulatory diagnostic services or home or nursing care? Is all the increase in hospitalization medically justified? A more detailed study of the Medicare experience and better methods of evaluating health services will be necessary to answer these questions.

Maldistribution and unequal access

The relationship between urban residence and health services is difficult to summarize, but certain points stand out. First, the geographic distribution of health workers and facilities is spotty and unplanned. Second, people not only have unequal access to services because of financial barriers, but also because of limitations related to race, age, education, and other factors.

The concentration of health workers and large hospitals in major cities makes ambulatory services more readily available to local residents. The effect of proximity is most evident in terms of physician and dental visits. The inner city poor, on the other hand, have paradoxically high rates of physician visits, but they do not use physicians for pediatric or preventive care as much as the rest of the population does. In spite of a recent strong trend toward increased use of emergency rooms and urban hospital outpatient departments, private practitioners still provide the bulk of ambulatory care in cities, as elsewhere.

The heaviest use of hospitals is found in the relatively small hospitals of towns and smaller cities. In larger cities, the very poor and the affluent have better access to hospitals than do residents with marginal incomes. Non-whites are at a disadvantage in terms of access to both physicians and hospitals, and this disadvantage is not entirely the result of poverty. Urban residents are more likely to have hospital and surgical insurance. Recent changes in the use of hospitals following the introduction of Medicare indicate that there has been and probably still remains an unmet need for health services in certain segments of the population. The question of whether hospital services are used excessively in some places and by some providers cannot be clearly resolved in the absence of uniform records. The predominant method of financing health care, that of insurance against surgical and hospital costs, with little provision for ambulatory and home care, has created a situation in which there is minimum restraint on the overuse of hospitals.

IMPROVING ACCESS

Social justice requires that we set as our objective equal access to good health services for all, not determined by ability to pay.

This is an internationally recognized objective for urban health services, affirmed by an Expert Committee of the World Health Organization in 1963,[28] which also stipulated that services should be comprehensive and subject to continuous evaluation and adaptation and that the public should participate in planning and operation.

What are the chances of obtaining such an elevated objective?

Organization and management

The state of our urban health services is like that of an old-fashioned machine shop in which a number of transmission belts are missing. Much of the necessary machinery is in place, and some of it is functioning smoothly. Several elements, however, are disconnected from the source of economic power and lie idle or function inefficiently. The whole apparatus has been put together piecemeal over a long period of time, and there never was a blueprint.

Clearly, a plan is the first requirement. Some halting steps in the direction of planning comprehensive urban health services were taken under the authority of the 1966 Partnership for Health Act, which established state and local comprehensive health planning agencies and began the difficult task of coordinating the planning functions of numerous pre-existing private and voluntary agencies. At the same time, the picture was confused by new laws establishing Regional Medical Programs, originally intended to deal with the leading causes of death (heart disease, cancer, and stroke) but undergoing changes in the writing and administration of the law. These agencies will now be merged with Comprehensive Health Planning Agencies and succeeded by regional Health Systems Agencies (National Health Planning and Resources Development Act of 1974, PL 93-641). Still, planning authority is spread out among state and local governments, federally funded programs, and multiple private and public hospitals, clinics, and other organizations.[29] Clear-cut plans, linking ambulatory and hospital care at all levels of complexity, will probably not become practicable until a more uniform system of financing health care can be established to make it possible for planning to be connected with budgeting and the authority to allocate money in accordance with agreed-upon priorities.

Today we appear to lack two fundamentals for effective planning: a national health policy and the underlying consensus that good health care is a right of every citizen. That consensus has been achieved, not only in socialist countries, but also in most Western industrial nations.[30] Because of its fundamental importance, we will deal with this issue at greater length in Chapter 8. But first, there are some intermediate managerial and technical steps to be taken to prepare the way. These include planning and organization of individual elements of the system, the training and efficient use of health manpower, and the development of methods of quality control. The first two subjects will be discussed in this chapter and the third in Chapter 6.

Large urban health centers can take advantage of a businesslike managerial approach. Most have grown by accretion and merger for the same reasons that businesses have grown: efficiency, a greater and more powerful mass of capital, and economies of scale. It is obviously more convenient and practicable to have a maternity hospital, a children's hospital, and a general hospital with associated services together on the same site and under a single management than to have them scattered about the city wherever interested parties first organized them. This process has not been carried to the point of maximum benefit. In large cities and, particularly, in small cities and towns, the merger of small and inefficient hospitals, along with related planning for transportation to maintain contact with the patient population, offers unmistakable advantages. The main obstacles are local pride and political fragmentation, particularly that associated with the social polarization of central city and suburban populations.

But even large urban hospital services are notoriously unbusinesslike in many respects. The difficulties stem from several sources. A key problem is that the output of the health industry is services rather than goods, and a peculiarly difficult kind of service to measure and evaluate at that. The recent shift of a large part of national health expenditures from the private to the public sector following the enactment of Medicare and Medicaid has thrust upon public attention some of the managerial failures of our health care system. Unequal access is a basic defect we have already documented in some detail. What alarms the public most is the apparently limitless skyrocketing of hospital and other health care costs.[31] An outcry, loud enough to obscure most other issues, has gone up for cost control.

One response to this outcry has been to look for health care models in which some control has been achieved. The system of prepaid group practice, which originated during World War II to serve the employees of the Kaiser Corporation has attracted much attention. Its outstanding achievement has been a proven ability to reduce hospital use by its members to 60 percent of that experienced by fellow workers under different systems of payment. Kaiser has been able to do this because it can regulate both ambulatory and hospital use in a single system with a planned budget. "Health maintenance organizations" have recently been recommended by the Administration and by Congress, modeled in general on the Kaiser Program. Experienced Kaiser managers caution, however, that the success of the system depends upon careful adherence to a "genetic code" with six essential features:

1. Prepayment
2. Group practice
3. A medical center (i.e., control of both ambulatory and hospital services)
4. Voluntary enrollment
5. Capitation payment (i.e., physicians and hospitals are paid according to the number enrolled in the program, not according to individual services)
6. Comprehensive coverage (i.e., all necessary services are provided)[32, 33]

Other advantages claimed for prepaid systems, such as better preventive practice, more rational work allocation, and increased subscriber satisfaction, are plausible because of the high degree of managerial control but have not been so clearly demonstrated as financial efficiency. One study of the Health Insurance Plan of New York (HIP) does suggest that enrollment in this prepaid system is associated with lower rates of prematurity, perinatal mortality, and possibly, with lower general mortality among the aged.[34] Prepaid groups, such as Kaiser, HIP, and the Group Health Cooperative of Puget Sound, operate in large cities where blocks of employees and other subscribers can be recruited. Much of the strength of these groups can be attributed to the fact that they have enrolled mainly middle-class subscribers with stable incomes. Whether the system will function equally well with poorer people whose premiums must be paid by public funds is being tested in Oregon and elsewhere. Preliminary reports suggest that removing the cost barrier tends to equalize the use of health services by indigent and self-supporting populations.[35]

The Kaiser program has given a valuable demonstration of the fact that better overall management of health services can control costs, though its own advocates doubt that it can be extended to serve the entire population. For those who can afford to join, access is probably better and costs are definitely more predictable, but many Americans can pay for Kaiser no more readily than they can pay for private care.

Neighborhood health centers were introduced as programs of social reform rather than as experiments in managerial change, and we shall consider their politically significant story in Chapter 8. At this point, however, it should be noted that the more successful centers, by planning and feedback evaluation of their services, have been able to render ambulatory services of a quality comparable to that of other established providers of health care.[36] In terms of access, these centers have been instrumental in bringing services to some badly underserved areas, though the numbers of people they have been able to reach are small. The Nixon Administration's decision to eliminate the Office of Economic Opportunity in 1973 put the neighborhood health centers in desperate financial straits.

A strong movement is now under way in this country toward more rational allocation of the work of health care. Pediatricians were the first among the specialists to acknowledge the fact that they were not working efficiently. The practicing pediatrician is overtrained for the work of well-baby care, which constitutes the bulk of his practice. Similar examples immediately come to mind in obstetrics, internal medicine, and surgery. Not only are highly trained experts spending too much of their time on simple, repetitive work, but nurses, nurses' aides, and others are also wasting their skills on clerical and other tasks for which they have not been prepared and which others, with more suitable training, could do better. The unplanned development of health manpower has produced a system that, far from being the shapeless "non-system" it is sometimes called, is in fact a rigid, hierarchical structure.

The education of health workers has been selected as a point at which change might be introduced. A new breed of health workers, specifically trained to "expand" the work of the physician, should make new and more efficient work patterns possible. The training of physicians' assistants, begun by Estes at Duke in 1965, and of nurse practitioners, following Silver's initial program at Colorado, started a process that is gathering momentum.[37] The introduction of new workers, by itself, however, will be of limited value unless there are related changes in the delivery system as well as in education. Such changes are more feasible in planned and organized systems like Kaiser or the neighborhood health centers than in the solo fee-for-service pattern in which the practitioner has little time or training to improve the management of his practice.

Group practice, prepayment, and task-directed education for the rational allocation of work are promising developments. More individual groups and highly organized systems are emerging, though slowly and unevenly.

But will these technical developments in the delivery of health care bring more doctors into the ghettos or convert crowded and impersonal outpatient departments into convenient comprehensive care centers? Will more efficiency and better organization solve the problems of maldistribution and unequal access, which are the major difficulties confronting the city dweller trying to obtain health care?

We cannot answer "yes" to these questions until we can begin to see how these organizational and managerial methods can be connected to sources of economic energy. A good plan is certainly a prerequisite to better allocation of resources, both geographically and economically, but no plan will work without a flow of money. More efficient work distribution and hospital use can benefit consumers, but not if they cannot afford to buy into the system. Nurse practitioners and physicians' assistants may ultimately improve the distribution of primary care, but most of them will no more choose to work in an urban slum than most doctors choose to now, unless better pay and better working conditions obtain. Solving the problems of maldistribution and unequal access must ultimately depend upon more flexible, more manageable, and more equitable means of financing health care.

Paying for care

Self-payment. There are basically three methods of meeting health care costs in the United States: self-payment, categorical public payment, and social insurance. Self-payment, either direct or via private insurance, is the principal method of health care financing. From the end of World War II until 1965, private expenditures accounted for about 75 percent of the total national expenditures for health and medical care. Since Medicare and Medicaid, the private share has dropped to 62 percent. It has been possible to adhere to private financing to this extent only because of the forced-draft growth of private health insurance as a means of avoiding government health insurance. In 1940, private insurance benefits paid a negligible proportion of personal health care costs. By 1965, one-quarter of such costs were met in this way, with little change since then.[38]

The remarkable growth of nonprofit (Blue Cross and Blue Shield) and profit-making private health insurance in two decades (1940-1960) led many to hope that a universal system of financing could be based on private insurance. Recent proposals for "national" health insurance favored by the American Medical Association and the Nixon and Ford administrations have been based on extending private health insurance, either by federal subsidy of voluntary purchases, directly or through tax credits, or by requiring employers to purchase such insurance, with financing through a combination of payroll tax and direct subsidy. The concepts of prepayment and group practice in "Health Maintenance Organizations" have been linked to some of these proposals, but the fundamental method of financing remains self-payment.

There are several reasons to doubt that such an approach will get at the root problems of unequal access and maldistribution. Two points stand out. First is the probability that any system of voluntary insurance will fail to cover precisely those people who are most in need of care. At the time Medicare was passed, the insurance industry itself supported the new law, since it recognized that it could not sell adequate coverage at acceptable premiums to the elderly, who constitute a high-need, low-income group. Even if funds were furnished and some degree of compulsion (such as requiring employers to buy insurance) were introduced, many of the people most in need of health services would continue to be the least likely to be covered: the poor and those with marginal incomes, their children, the physically or mentally disabled, and racial and ethnic minorities. As voluntary insurance was unable to cover all persons, so it has proven to be incapable of financing all services. Major omissions in every policy are long-term care of the seriously disabled and almost all treatment for mental illness. There are strong indications that the limits of private health insurance have been reached in this country.

A second serious drawback to a national health program based on the purchase of individual or group insurance is that the administrative authority necessary to cope with the problem of maldistribution of services would be absent in such a system or, at least, so diffused as to be ineffective. Furthermore, as with the matter of coverage, there would be no economic motive for private insurers to extend services into inner city or rural areas where needs are high and cash is short. Better distribution of services and equal access to them for all citizens should be high national priorities based on broad principles of social justice. They will not be achieved without some social cost in money and in the hitherto largely unrestrained professional privilege of health care providers to offer what services they wish, wherever they wish, and on their own terms. Here, in the impending necessity for regulation of the activities of physicians, hospitals, and other members of the system, lies the main resistance to a national health service. More will be said on this subject in Chapter 8 when we consider prospects for federally administered national health insurance.

Categorical Public Payment. Public funds (federal, state, and local) expended for health-related functions can be roughly subdivided into two classes: categorical and social insurance (Table

5.7). Categorical payments are made directly from federal funds to persons who can demonstrate that they belong to the defined group, with no requirement for prior contribution. The list of categorical programs is a miscellaneous one which has grown by accretion since the establishment of the U.S. Marine Hospital Service in 1798. New programs were established as wars and movements for social and economic reform brought the health needs of certain classes of citizens to public attention. The categories served by these programs vary from broad social groupings (all public school children) to highly specific classes (blind or low-income residents of a specific area). The services provided may be essentially complete, as for persons in active military service and their dependents, but are more often limited to specific kinds of care (well-baby care, but not care for illness; care for service-connected disability, but not for other illnesses). These restrictions on type of service are the source of much confusion and resentment among both consumers and providers of health services. Much of the effort of medical social work is expended in searching for an appropriate category into which a particular patient can be fitted and on assembling the evidence needed to prove that he is entitled to the services.

Even more confining are the financial limitations of most public programs for providing health services. The "means test," which has been imposed on recipients of public funds for health care, is a requirement that an individual apply for services or for payment and present evidence that he is a legitimate applicant and cannot afford to pay for the service without public assistance. In short, he must beg for help. Criteria of eligibility vary widely. The largest single program, Medicaid, has introduced complex payment formulas, borrowed from the insurance industry, which require recipients to pay part of the costs themselves by means of deductibles, "co-insurance," and maximum limits.

Constraints on the amount of service to which an individual is "entitled" by reason of his membership in a particular category can clearly become a barrier to access. Poor people often lack the cash to pay deductibles. A patient may have to leave a nursing home at the end of an arbitrary number of days regardless of need. A diabetic with multiple complications requiring repeated

Table 5.7
Expenditures for health services and supplies from all public sources, United States (1972-1973)

	Amount (millions of dollars)	*Public Expenditures (%)*
EXPENDITURES FOR SPECIAL CATEGORIES OF PERSONS		
Public assistance (vendor medical payments, including Medicaid)	8,923.1	26.2
Defense Department hospital and medical care (including military dependents)	2,597.0	7.6
Veterans hospital and medical care	2,587.3	7.6
General hospital and medical care (mainly mental hospitals)	5,049.9	14.9
Maternal and child health services	455.3	1.3
School health	320.0	0.9
Other public health activities	2,810.7	8.3
Medical vocational rehabilitation	197.2	0.6
Office of Economic Opportunity	152.4	0.5
TOTAL	23,092.9	67.9
SOCIAL INSURANCE		
Health insurance for the aged (Medicare)	9,478.0	27.9
Workmen's compensation (medical)	1,370.0	4.0
Temporary disability insurance (medical)	68.2	0.2
TOTAL	10,916.2	32.1
GRAND TOTAL PUBLIC EXPENDITURES	34,009.1	100.0

Source: B. S. Cooper, N. L. Worthington, and P. A. Piro, National Health Expenditures, 1929-73. *Social Security Bulletin,* February, 1974, Table 3.

hospital admissions may be impoverished if he is not initially old enough or disabled enough to be "eligible." These restrictions have been imposed in order to limit costs and the extent of public liability. Cost restraints imposed on the consumer, however, are unlikely to be effective in a system in which the use of services is strongly influenced, if not largely controlled, by providers. The unavailable doctor, or the doctor who orders weekly vitamin "shots," the hospital with a long waiting list, or the hospital with empty beds, probably influence the use and cost of services more than do individual decisions to seek or defer care based on an awareness of cost. Undoubtedly such constraints do prevent some people from using services under some circumstances.

But the very existence of such barriers to access raises a larger question. Should the decision to seek care ever be determined by cost? Faced with a life-threatening illness, most people choose to disregard cost, whether they can afford to or not. When the illness is minor or of unknown seriousness, a cost barrier is at least as likely to inhibit early detection and treatment as it is to prevent unnecessary use of services. At the same time, another economic mechanism, the fee-for-service method of payment, tends to make it profitable for the physician to increase the number of visits made by each patient and to admit patients more frequently to the hospital. The physician's advice, rather than the patient's preference, is the main determinant of frequency of use of services once the initial contact has been made. On balance, then, the categorical system of spending public money for health care, by individual units of service, with limitations of eligibility and enforced cost-sharing, has not only failed to limit costs but may actually encourage high rates of use. International comparisons suggest that the system in the United States does in fact operate this way, since per capita physician visits are twice as frequent in the United States as in Sweden.[39] The effort to control health care costs by placing financial obstacles in the way of the patient, rather than by regulating the providers, is not only ineffectual, but a bad social bargain as well, since it hinders prevention and early treatment and leads to greater ultimate costs.

Categorical public programs that provide more comprehensive health services, as in the military and the Veterans' Administration, have by and large eliminated both economic barriers to use and the stimulus to overuse arising from the fee-for-service system, since the hospitals are government-regulated and the providers salaried. The recipients of service appear to be somewhat more satisfied than those recipients who obtain services through other types of categorical program, if only because financial threats and constraints are alleviated. Whether costs are effectively controlled within such a system is difficult to determine because of the differences in the populations served and in the methods of cost accounting between military and veterans' services on the one hand and private and other civilian services on the other. Theoretically, a government-owned and government-controlled system should be more manageable, though effective incentives for cost control are probably lacking at the present time in both systems.

Social Insurance. The introduction of Medicare in 1965 seemed to many physicians an unprecedented step toward socialization. The fact is that the principle of social insurance was established in this country as long ago as 1908, when a federal act established limited benefits for designated classes of public employees. Workmen's compensation laws were passed first in Wisconsin in 1911.[40] The system has been extended subsequently to all states, but coverage is not uniform. For example, the laws are compulsory in only one-half of the states, and benefits are limited in amount or duration in 12 jurisdictions.[41] Social insurance payments differ from categorical payments in that they are made from a special fund created by compulsory contributions from workers or employers. Benefits under Medicare and workmen's compensation are held to be an earned legal right, deriving from the payment of taxes, specified by law, and enforceable in the courts. As noted in the previous chapter, the funding of Medicare is really a transfer of funds rather than an insurance program in which benefits arise from the individual's own contribution. The same may be said of workmen's compensation. But both programs depend upon special contributions, as taxes or premiums from employer or employee. In the eyes of the public, they are insurance programs, and the benefits are validated by having been earned.

Social health insurance, therefore, despite years of bitter opposition, is expanding in the United States and is remarkably well accepted as long as it is presented as an earned right rather than as public assistance. The expansion has been brought about mainly by legislation extending the Social Security law to cover not only the health care of the aged, but disability benefits for physical or mental impairment and for dependents and survivors as well. Workmen's compensation benefits have also been expanding to a point at which they have begun to resemble sickness insurance, as a result of increasingly broad interpretations by courts and compensation authorities of what disabilities can be considered related to occupation. Again, the trend indicates that extensive social insurance is acceptable in this country as long as it can be made respectable by some connection, however tenuous, with work.

More and broader programs of social insurance will probably result from present trends. Uniform National Health Insurance would significantly improve access to health services, particularly for those with marginal incomes for whom direct payment for health care looms as a large expense. Recent experience in Quebec supports this prediction.[42] Social insurance, confined to financing alone, however, would neither regulate costs nor bring about a redistribution of services. The equitable provision of adequate funds and the establishment of a national administrative framework are essential steps toward dealing with these problems, but their solution will require planning and administration at a level not now possible. Before we proceed to describe the necessary features of a National Health Service, however, let us take a look at how those who can afford the present costs obtain their health care.

SUBURBAN HEALTH

6

In the 1920's, the streetcar and the mass-produced automobile opened up the city. Urban Americans were nostalgic for the countryside. With pleasure, they discovered that they could now own a house with some land around it and still work in town. The suburbs flourished in the United States in particular because, by the late nineteenth century, the intense industrial development of the inner cities had made them unattractive places to live, whereas the area around the city was sparsely populated, and land was cheap. The suburbs became a refuge, a home, and a symbol of achievement. The good life, most middle-class citizens of mid-century America expected, was to be found there.

Since World War II, however, doubts have arisen. For the individual, suburban life too often proves monotonous, fragmented, and empty. As a social mechanism, the suburb seems to have been transformed from an escape route for the inner city dweller into a racially exclusive ring that locks him in. A small but growing countercurrent of population movement back into renewed sections of some older cities is detectable. Another new trend is the outward movement of light manufacturing and retail sales into the suburbs, attracted by increased population, lower taxes, and less expensive land. Single houses in the peripheral community are coming to be mixed with shopping centers, apartment houses, small factories, and recreational areas rather than with farms, while new waves continue to expand urban sprawl concentrically to the point where neighboring cities flow together into conurbations.

Nevertheless, the suburbs still look good to most Americans. The dynamic growth that began in the 1920's continued steadily through the 1960's. About 1968 we crossed a watershed, when the suburbs replaced farms and small towns as the place where the largest segment of the population lives.

The attractions of the suburbs are evident and familiar. They have continued to grow at the expense of non-metropolitan regions, and, since World War II, partially at the expense of inner cities as well, because they offer more space for living, greater safety, and more congenial surroundings. Also, it is generally assumed that life is healthier in the suburbs.

The purpose of this chapter is to question this assumption, as we are questioning everything else about middle-class America. Is suburban life really healthier than life in the central city, and how does it compare with small town and rural life? Is the quality of suburban health related to the quality of health services, or is it merely a by-product of suburban social and economic factors? And finally, what lessons learned from the suburban experience can be applied to our efforts to improve health in the nation as a whole?

THE QUALITY OF HEALTH IN SUBURBIA

The suburbs dominate the residential pattern in the United States today, and they have now existed long enough that two sizable generations have never lived anywhere else. Do these native suburbanites live a healthy life?

Ironically, there is little objective information with which to answer this question. Health in the inner city has been studied, but suburban health has been taken for granted. For example, reports on morbidity and use of services from the National Health Survey combine the suburbs with the central cities. A few clues can be found in mortality data, which is subdivided by central city and non-central city metropolitan counties. The counties that can be considered suburban (metropolitan but not central city) in this classification are contiguous to the central city and related to it by being essentially metropolitan in character and socially and economically integrated with it. Some farmland remains, but it is rapidly giving way to the bulldozer and the automobile. This is the suburban fringe–scarcely rural any longer, and not yet fully urban. These counties, compared with the central city and non-metropolitan counties, have intermediate population densities. In Table 6.1 the suburbs are shown as subdivisions of the metropolitan (SMSA) counties, with the inner ring of suburbs consisting of "other urban" (2,500 to 50,000 population) and the outer ring designated as (metropolitan) "rural farm and non-farm." Some farmlands are included in such geographically large SMSA as Los Angeles, since the SMSA's are made up of counties, and some counties are very extensive, especially in the Southwest (Appendix A).

Here in the suburbs are found the highest proportions of the rich, the young, and the highly educated and the lowest proportions of the poor, the non-white, and the elderly (Table 6.1). Given these statistics, it seems likely that individuals who live in these counties will have the best health of any group in the country.

Longer lives

Mortality rates strongly support this idea. Though the suburbs are not far from metropolitan areas where many factors combine to increase mortality rates from cancer, heart disease, and other major causes, at least 37 percent of deaths in the United States are attributed to causes for which the lowest mortality rates are found in the non-central city (suburban) counties. The lowest average age-adjusted death rates in the country are found in the suburban counties: 7.6 percent below non-metropolitan counties and 9.0 percent below central city rates (Fig. 1.1).

Table 6.1
Social and economic characteristics of the U.S. population, by residence (1970)

	METROPOLITAN					*NON-METROPOLITAN*				
	Total	*Central Cities*	*Other Urban*	*Rural Non-farm*	*Rural Farm*	*Total*	*Urban*	*Rural Non-farm*	*Rural Farm*	*U.S. (total)*
Persons, percent	68.6	31.4	29.1	6.9	1.1	31.4	13.0	14.4	4.0	100
Persons per square mile	360	4,462		203		19.8				57.5
Median age (years)	28.0	28.8	27.4	26.3	31.4	28.3	28.0	27.7	32.2	28.1
Persons under 18 years, percent	34.1	31.9	35.5	38.4	35.5	35.0	32.8	36.7	36.0	34.4
Persons 65 years and over, percent	9.3	10.8	8.0	7.6	10.4	11.3	11.7	11.1	10.5	9.9
Non-white, percent	13.5	22.5	5.9	5.9		10.4	10.2	10.5		12.5
Public assistance recipients, percent	5.2	7.2	3.5	3.7	3.0	5.6	5.2	6.4	3.9	5.3
Median family income ($1,000)	10.5	9.5	11.6	10.0	9.1	7.8	8.6	7.5	6.8	9.6
Persons with 4 years high school education or more, percent	55.3	50.8	61.5	51.7	45.9	45.9	52.1	41.7	41.2	52.3
Persons with 4 years college education or more, percent	12.0	10.9	14.2	9.3	6.1	7.7	10.5	6.2	4.2	10.7

Source: U.S. Bureau of Census, *1970 Census,* PC(1)-A1 and PC(1)-B1.

Less infectious disease

One reason for these differences is that the chances of dying of infectious disease are minimal in suburban counties. Influenza and pneumonia, which produce higher mortality outside of cities and in central cities, produce the lowest mortality in the suburbs (Fig. 1.2). Several other acute infectious diseases with relatively high urban mortality, including streptococcal, diphtherial, and meningococcal infections, also tend to show lower suburban death rates, though, remarkably, deaths from these diseases are now so few that the figures are not statistically significant. Aggregate death rates from all infectious diseases other than syphilis and tuberculosis again show a distinct advantage for the suburban counties (Fig. 6.1). Morbidity data for acute infectious diseases, which would include much larger numbers, are not reported separately for the suburbs.

Tuberculosis, which has been associated with industrial cities for generations, continues to kill proportionately more people within the cities of the United States than elsewhere (Chapter 2). The advantage of suburban residence is clearly shown in the lowest mortality rates for this disease (Fig. 1.2).[1] In Boston, Cleveland, New York, Philadelphia, and San Francisco, rates of infection are markedly lower in the suburbs than in the central cities, as indicated by the prevalence of positive tuberculin reactors among Navy recruits.[2] Even in the central county of a metropolitan area, such as Cleveland, rates of new active cases of tuberculosis have remained 50 percent higher within the city limits than for the county as a whole.[3]

High rates of disease and death due to tuberculosis have repeatedly been shown to be associated with foreign birth and residence, poverty, crowded and inadequate housing, and contact with active cases and, probably by secondary association, with non-white races.[4, 5] All of these environmental and personal factors are more prevalent in central cities than in the suburban fringe and go far to explain the observed differences.

Another reason for lower tuberculosis death rates in the suburbs, however, may be the quality and availability of diagnostic and treatment services. Since the introduction of streptomycin in

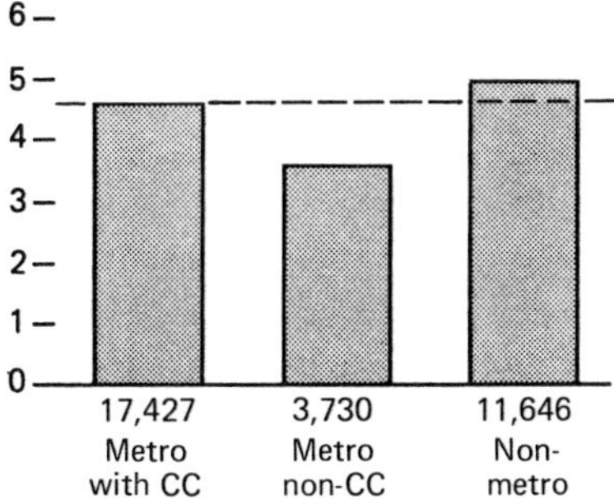

Fig. 6.1 **Deaths attributed to infective and parasitic diseases other than tuberculosis and syphilis** (ICDA 000-009, 020-089, 098-136): age-adjusted annual mortality rates (U.S.), 1969–1971, by county of residence. (Cf. Fig. 1.1 and Appendix B, Table 3.)

1947, and other effective antituberculous drugs subsequently, the prevalence of the disease has dropped to low enough levels that mass X-ray screening has become a very expensive method of detection.[6] Among other reasons for its cost, X-ray screening offered on a voluntary basis tends to be most used by middle-class persons who have the lowest disease rates.[7] This fact suggests that suburban residents are more likely to have the disease detected at an early and more treatable stage.

Fragmentary evidence, therefore, points to the likelihood that the suburban resident is less often exposed to infectious disease. If he does become infected, he is also more likely to have it detected promptly and to obtain earlier access to effective treatment.

Safer appendicitis

Common surgical conditions may also be less dangerous for the suburban population than for others. The incidence of appendicitis is evidently declining in the United States.[8] Though diet, use of laxatives, and parasitic infections have been suggested as causes of the disease, there is no good evidence that they influence the rates observed in the United States, which appear to be decreasing broadly in both metropolitan and rural areas.[9] Early diagnosis and prompt intervention, on the other hand, have been

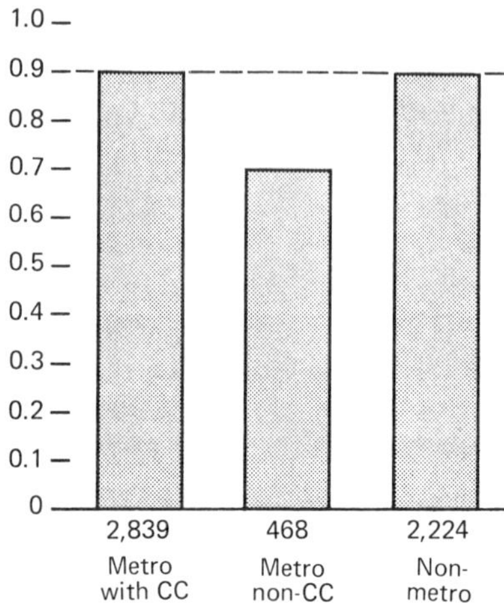

Fig. 6.2 **Deaths attributed to appendicitis** (ICDA 7th Revision 550-553): age-adjusted annual mortality rates (U.S.), 1959–1961, by county of residence. (Cf. Fig. 1.1 and Appendix B, Table 29; data are not available for 1969–1971.)

credited with a 90 percent reduction in mortality between 1940 and 1960. Differences in mortality rates from appendicitis, therefore, probably reflect differences in the quality and availability of surgical and, perhaps, antibiotic treatment. Figure 6.2 shows that deaths from appendicitis occurred in suburban counties, in 1960, at rates more than 20 percent below the rates for both central cities and non-metropolitan counties. The relationship between this finding and prompt treatment is brought out by a study of appendicitis in Cleveland in 1946. Though the authors interpreted their findings cautiously, the data suggest that higher economic levels (measured as rents and rent equivalents, by census tracts) are correlated with lower mortality, with a lower proportion of cases complicated by peritonitis and abscess, with fewer median hours of delay, and with fewer anesthetic deaths.[10] The poorer economic areas, of course, are mainly in the central city, and the wealthier in the peripheral suburbs.

Death rates from peptic ulcer are probably also influenced by the promptness and adequacy of treatment for the major complications, which are hemorrhage, perforation, and obstruction. As with appendicitis, death from this cause is less frequent in the suburban counties than elsewhere (Fig. 6.3).

Lower maternal and infant mortality

Childbirth is also less dangerous to the suburban mother and her infant than to mothers and infants elsewhere. The chances of a woman's dying during pregnancy in the United States have been reduced 95 percent over the past 35 years. A progressive extension of prenatal services and an increase in the use of hospitals for deliveries are the principal reasons for this great achievement.[11] Modern obstetrical care, like many other advances in health care, was initially developed in urban hospitals, and for years metropolitan maternal mortality ratios were lower than those elsewhere. In the last decade, however, the gap between metropolitan and non-metropolitan counties has narrowed greatly (Table 6.2). This difference, in 1960, could be attributed mainly to high rates of death from toxemia and hemorrhage among non-metropolitan women. Since these complications of pregnancy can

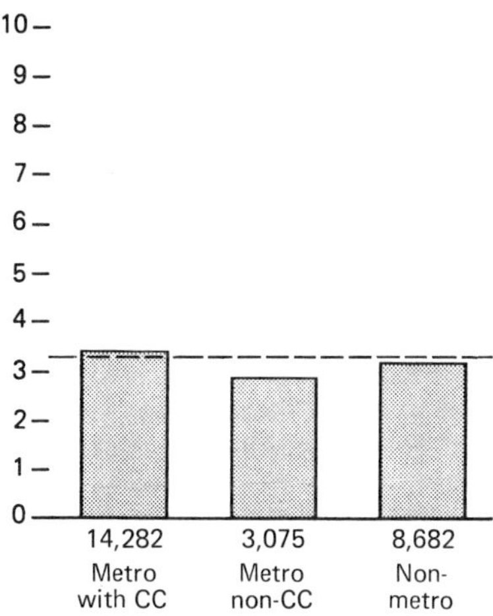

Fig. 6.3 **Deaths attributed to peptic ulcer** (ICDA 531-533): age-adjusted annual mortality rates (U.S.), 1969–1971, by county of residence. (Cf. Fig. 1.1 and Appendix B, Table 20.)

Table 6.2
Maternal mortality ratios, United States (1960 and 1969)

	Metropolitan Counties	*Non-Metropolitan Counties*	*Difference (% of metropolitan)*
Deaths from complications of pregnancy, etc. (ICD, 7th Rev., 640-689) per 100,000 live births, 1960	33.0	44.3	34.2
Deaths from complications of pregnancy, etc. (ICD, 8th Rev., 630–678), per 100,000 live births, 1969	21.5	23.7	10.2

Source: *Vital Statistics of the U.S., 1960* (Washington, D.C.: Government Printing Office, 1963), Vol. 2, Part A, Table 1-Z; *Ibid, 1969,* Vol. 2, Part B, Table 7-9 and Vol. 1, Table 1-56.

be recognized and managed more safely with skilled prenatal and obstetrical care, it is probable that the reduction of metropolitan/non-metropolitan differences has been achieved mainly by improved services.

Similarly, infant mortality has been reduced almost 65 percent during the past 35 years. "Advances in medicine, the expansion and improvement of health facilities, the greater availability of medical and other health personnel, and aggressive action by public and private health and welfare agencies contributed to these declines in mortality," according to a recent definitive review of the subject.[12]

Infants born in metropolitan areas have a better chance of surviving to their first birthdays than do those born in non-metropolitan counties (Table 6.3). Mortality ratios in the first month after birth are similar, but the risk is distinctly greater for non-metropolitan infants between one month and one year of age. The gap between metropolitan and non-metropolitan ratios has been significantly reduced over the past decade.

As in other industrialized nations, infant mortality in the United States fell steadily after the late nineteenth century. A leveling-off of the decline took place in the 1950's, however, and it began to fall behind those declines seen in other Western countries.[13, 14] Concern over this development has led to more intensive studies of infant mortality.

It is now clear that within major cities of the United States there are sizable poor populations in which infant mortality is 50 to 100 percent higher than in more affluent sections of the same city.[15]

Within metropolitan counties, higher educational levels achieved by the parents and higher family incomes are both associated (apparently independently) with lower infant mortality ratios.[16] Though maternal and infant mortality ratios for suburban coun-

Table 6.3
Infant mortality ratios, United States (1960 and 1970)

	Metropolitan Counties	*Non-metropolitan Counties*	*Difference (% of metropolitan)*
Infant mortality (under 1 year, per 1,000 live births), 1960	24.9	28.0	12.4
Infant mortality (under 1 year, per 1,000 live births), 1970	19.5	21.2	8.7
Neonatal mortality (under 28 days, per 1,000 live births), 1960	18.6	18.9	1.6
Neonatal mortality (under 28 days, per 1,000 live births), 1970	14.8	15.6	5.4
Postneonatal mortality (28 days to 1 year, per 1,000 live births), 1960	6.3	10.1	60.3
Postneonatal mortality (28 days to 1 year, per 1,000 live births), 1970	4.7	5.6	19.1

Source: *Vital Statistics of the U.S., 1960* (Washington, D.C., U.S. Government Printing Office, 1963), Vol. 2, Part B, Table 9-2; *Ibid, 1970,* Vol. 2, Part B, Table 7-2 (1974).

ties are nowhere reported separately from those of central cities, it is clear that in order to produce the relatively favorable ratios reported for metropolitan areas as a whole, suburban ratios must be lower than both those in central cities and those in nonmetropolitan counties.

Social and environmental factors contribute to these differences in several ways. A high risk of infant mortality is associated with low birth weight (2,500 grams or less), which in turn is more frequent among births to parents of lower social and economic status. Other important risk factors are low social and economic status (independent of birth weight), illegitimacy, older parents, and large family size.[17]

The quantity and quality of health care received by mother and infant have an important effect on infant mortality, one which can be distinguished from the effect of social, economic, and biological conditions. A detailed study of all infant births and deaths in New York City in 1968 shows that only one-quarter of the women were judged to have received adequate health services as measured by a three-factor index (time of first prenatal visit, number of prenatal visits, and hospital service, whether ward or private). Furthermore, services were grossly misallocated. Among the 22,000 black and Puerto Rican mothers at social risk, less than 2 percent had adequate care. In each of four maternal risk groups and in each of four ethnic groups, more adequate care was found to be associated with lower rates of "prematurity" (low birth weight) and with lower infant mortality. If all women had had the pregnancy outcome of those receiving adequate health services, more than a thousand additional infants would have survived in a single year in New York City.[18]

Starting in the late 1960's and continuing at least through 1974, infant mortality in the United States again began to decline.[19] One important factor in the resumption of this interrupted trend probably was the refocusing of attention on improved services through planned maternal and infant care.

The advantage of urban residence for infants is particularly evident in lower rates of death from infectious diseases, birth injuries, and accidents.[20] In particular, in the suburban population infant mortality due to complications of pregnancy and childbirth

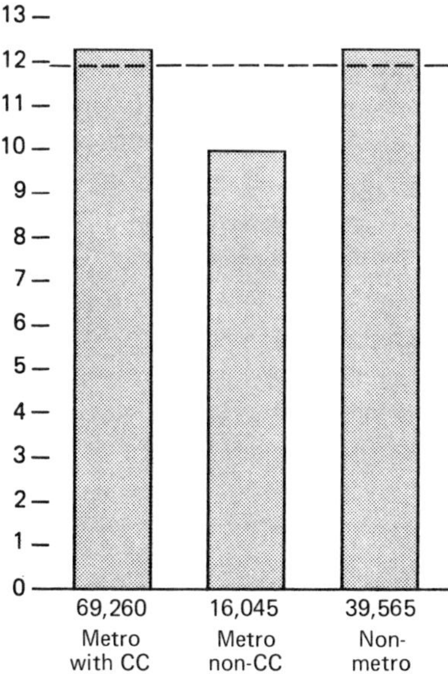

Fig. 6.4 **Deaths attributed to certain causes of mortality related to pregnancy and childbirth** (ICDA 760-769.2, 759.4-772, 774-778): age-specific annual mortality rates for infants of 1 year and under (U.S.), 1969–1971, by county of residence. (Cf. Fig. 1.1 and Appendix B, Table 24.)

is strikingly lower (Fig. 6.4). The specific example of tetanus illustrates how improved obstetrical practice can reduce the death rate. Infection and death due to tetanus are more frequent in nonmetropolitan areas today. A large proportion of deaths due to tetanus occur among newborn infants in rural areas where untrained midwives may still apply unsterilized dressings to the umbilical stump.[21]

Deaths attributed to congenital anomalies are also relatively less frequent in the suburban counties than elsewhere, probably because suburban infants have earlier and more adequate access to pediatric surgery and other supportive and rehabilitative services (Fig. 6.5).

In summary, women in metropolitan and suburban areas who enjoy social and economic advantages also face a minimal ob-

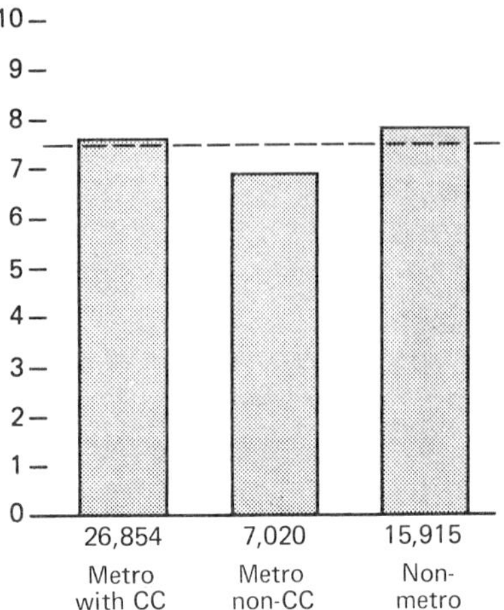

Fig. 6.5 **Deaths attributed to congenital anomalies** (ICDA 740-759): age-adjusted annual mortality rates (U.S.), 1969–1971, by county of residence. (Cf. Fig. 2.1 and Appendix B, Table 23).

stetrical risk, and their infants are more likely to survive the first year of life. Social status probably operates indirectly through better nutrition, education, and other supportive channels, but it favors the mother and child most directly by giving them access to better services.

Less chronic disability

Residence in the suburbs cannot prevent the onset of the major chronic disabling diseases, but it may mitigate their effects. Cancer and heart disease, as we have seen in Chapter 1, generally produce death rates that are inversely proportional to the distance of the area from urban centers. But there are exceptions to this rule, not only within these two categories of disease but among other types of chronic disabling disease as well. For a notable number of such conditions, mortality rates are significantly lower in suburban counties.

The few cancers for which mortality is lowest in the suburbs may reflect more accurate diagnosis and earlier treatment. Carcinoma of the cervix of the uterus, for example, causes 22 percent fewer deaths in suburban counties than elsewhere (Fig. 6.6). Evidence suggests, though it does not yet prove, that the use of cytological screening (the "Pap" test, 1940) has contributed to a 38 percent decline in deaths from this cause in the period 1950-1967.[22, 23, 24, 25] Furthermore, women in the top economic brackets tend to respond better to a screening program, whereas special efforts are needed to achieve comparable rates of use among those in the lowest economic groups.[26] Figure 6.6 could also be interpreted as representing more exposure to some causative factor, possibly infectious, which results in higher mortality rates from this cancer among poor women and those who marry and bear children at an early age.[27]

For certain major cardiovascular diseases, including hypertension, hypertensive heart disease, vascular disease of the central nervous system, and nephritis and nephrosis, age-adjusted mortality rates appear to be lower in suburban than in central city counties (Figs. 6.7 and 6.8). Non-metropolitan rates for these diseases, on the other hand, are generally high. The residential discrepancies are greatly reduced, however, when white and non-white

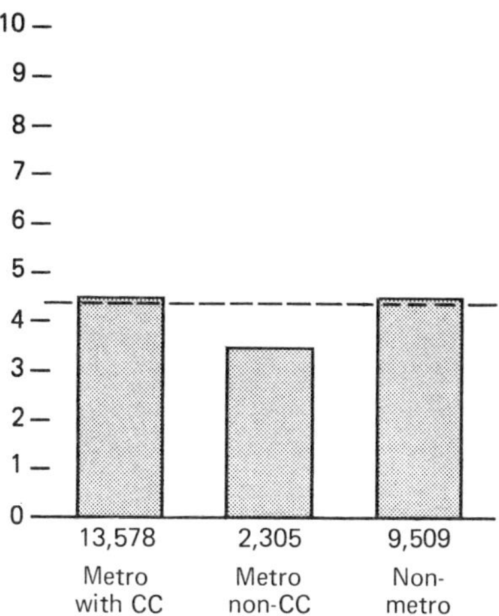

Fig. 6.6 **Deaths attributed to malignant neoplasm of cervix uteri** (ICDA 7th Revision 171): age-adjusted annual mortality rates (U.S.), 1959–1961, by county of residence. (Cf. Fig. 1.1 and Appendix B, Table 30; data are not available for 1969–1971.)

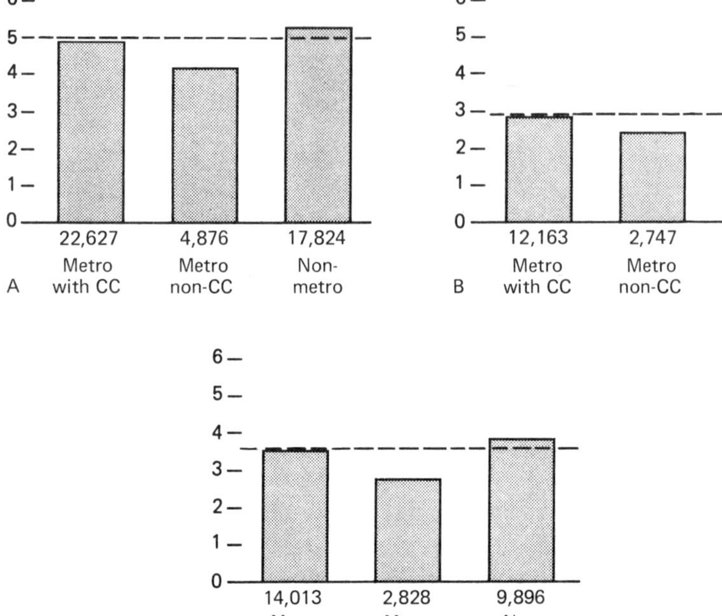

Fig. 6.7 **Deaths attributed to** (A) **hypertensive heart disease with or without renal disease** (ICDA 402, 404), (B) **hypertension** (ICDA 400, 401, 403), **and** (C) **nephritis and nephrosis** (ICDA 580-584): age-adjusted annual mortality rates (U.S.), 1969–1971, by county of residence. (Cf. Fig. 1.1 and Appendix B, Tables 14, 16, and 22.)

rates are examined separately. Hypertension, for unknown reasons, is highly associated with black racial origins. The prevalence of definite hypertension, for example, as determined in the National Health Examination, is 41.6 percent among black males in rural areas, compared with an expected rate of 27.5 percent for persons of the same age, sex, and race.[28] Race dominates the epidemiological picture. Modern methods of treating hypertension have been shown to prevent disability and death in controlled studies,[29, 30] but 1969-1971 mortality statistics fail to reveal any consistent differences in mortality by area of residence other than that which follows from the combination of high prevalence among blacks and the relative concentration of blacks in central cities and non-metropolitan areas. The effect of modern treatment on mortality should begin to become apparent soon, and it is likely to show up first in the suburban population.

Death attributed to diabetes is likely to be due to acute complications, such as diabetic acidosis or insulin shock, rather than to chronic complications, such as heart or kidney disease. When the latter occur, they are usually listed as the primary cause of death. The fact that diabetes mortality rates are distinctly lower in suburban areas again suggests better management of the dis-

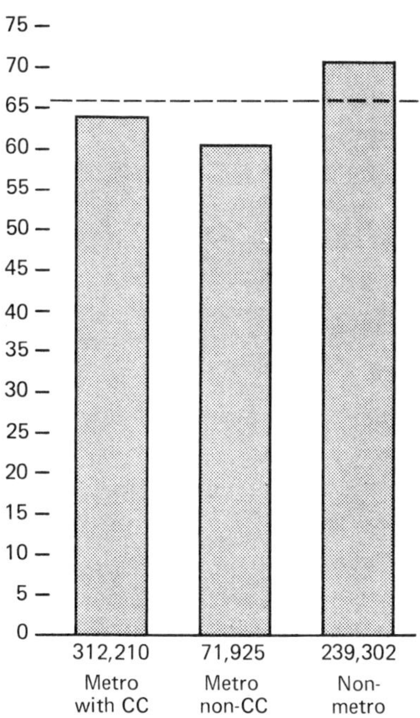

Fig. 6.8 **Deaths attributed to cerebrovascular disease** (ICDA 430-438): age-adjusted annual mortality rates (U.S.), 1969–1971, by county of residence. (Cf. Fig. 1.1 and Appendix B, Table 17.)

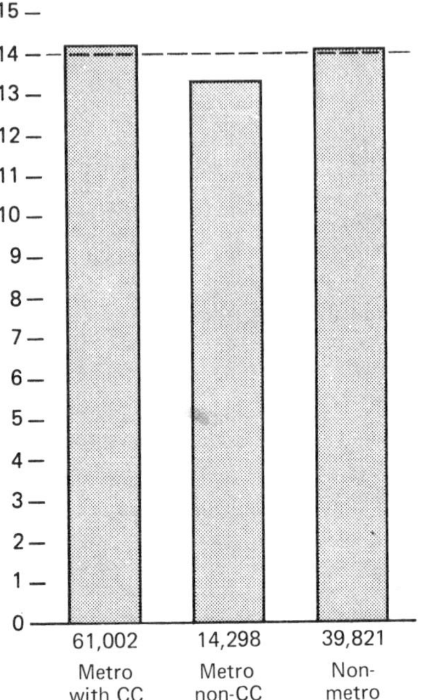

Fig. 6.9 **Deaths attributed to diabetes mellitus** (ICDA 250): age-adjusted annual mortality rates (U.S.), 1969–1971, by county of residence. (Cf. Fig. 1.1 and Appendix B, Table 11.)

ease and more prompt treatment of acute complications (Fig. 6.9).

Chronic pulmonary disease, because of its duration, is a major cause of disability, though it is less frequently a cause of death than cancer or heart disease. The lowest mortality rates for pulmonary tuberculosis and for pneumonia, which is frequently the terminal event in chronic disease of the respiratory system, have already been shown to occur in suburban counties (Fig. 1.2). Bronchitis, emphysema, and asthma also show definitely lower mortality rates in the suburbs (Fig. 6.10).

Though homicide and suicide are forms of sudden death, they

are often the outcome of severe emotional and social distress and probably reflect a much higher prevalence of emotional disability that does not end so dramatically. By far the lowest rates for both homicide and suicide are observed in suburban counties (Fig. 3.3). These differences probably express some of the social and economic advantages of suburban life, such as less crowding, less poverty, and better education, but they may also bear a relationship to the fact that middle- and upper-class persons with mental illness are more likely to receive prompt and individualized treatment and less likely to be confined for long periods in state mental hospitals or prisons.[32]

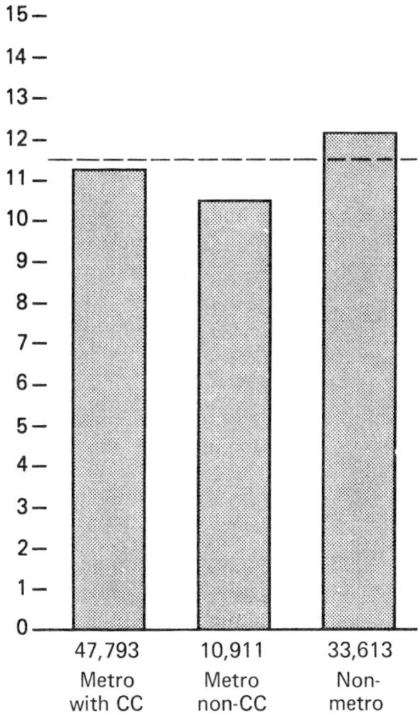

Fig. 6.10 **Deaths attributed to bronchitis, emphysema, and asthma** (ICDA 490-493): age-adjusted annual mortality rates (U.S.), 1969–1971, by county of residence. (Cf. Fig. 1.1 and Appendix B, Table 19.)

THE RELATIONSHIP BETWEEN SERVICES AND HEALTH

The rather spotty information on disease and death in the suburbs as distinct from other residential areas suggests that health services work to the advantage of suburban residents. But can we be sure that there are differences in the use of services related to residence?

The idea that suburban residents have better access to health services is supported by what evidence there is. Hospitalization rates in suburban counties are intermediate (Table 5.3b), but rates of physician and dental visits are relatively high (Table 5.3), and, for children under 17, they are higher than in any other residential area. Such a pattern suggests more preventive and health-maintenance care, with some avoidance of crisis hospitalization as a result.

Another way to estimate the suburbanites' access to health services is to examine how they differ from the rest of the population and then determine what these differences imply in the way of services. The suburbs have the highest income and educational levels and the lowest non-white population (Table 6.1). Higher income levels are associated with higher personal health expenditures[33] and with more frequent physician and dental visits.[34, 35] Lower proportions of non-white population, which here imply economic and social differences rather than differences associated with race as such, are also correlated with higher health expenditures and more access to physicians, dentists, and hospitals.[33, 34, 35, 36] Similarly, persons in the upper social classes have earlier access to individualized treatment for mental illness and are less likely to be hospitalized for long periods in public mental institutions.[32, 37]

Health professionals and specialized hospital services are concentrated in the large cities, but suburban residents probably find it easier to use these services than do inner city residents. Most suburban residents have private transportation, which readily overcomes the barrier of distance, and they also have more money and more health insurance, which are the keys to the system. In addition, physicians who provide primary and health maintenance care have their offices increasingly concentrated in the suburbs. In Boston in 1960, for example, socioeconomic class levels, as measured by income, education, and occupation, rise as one moves radially from the city center into the first ring of suburbs. The proportion of primary care (non-hospital-based) physicians also increases radially, from 56.2 per 100,000 population in the poor, central city areas, to 535.7 in the well-to-do western suburb of Brookline. Furthermore, this gap increased between 1940 and 1961. Since fewer than 20 percent of the primary physicians in the wealthier areas are general practitioners, it is evident that the internists, pediatricians, and obstetrician-gynecologists from whom the middle- and upper-class citizens of the United States obtain much of their primary care are increasingly located near paying patients in the suburban areas.[38, 39]

Good services and good health

One epidemiologist, now the Dean of a school of public health, while stressing the importance of air pollution and poverty as causes of mortality, minimized the effect of medical care thus: "The weight of evidence does not support the hypothesis that the health status of the population is largely dependent on the quality and quantity of its medical services . . . medical care is largely unrelated to the health status of the population."[40]

This statement, which expresses a point of view that is surprisingly prevalent among public health professionals, contradicts much of the evidence we have considered so far in this chapter, and the contradiction must be resolved. Priorities, planning, the allocation of resources, and the confidence with which we undertake to improve urban health depend heavily on whether we believe that providing more and better health services can in fact improve health.

Let us summarize the evidence. The relatively good state of health enjoyed by those who live in the suburbs depends to a significant extent on at least four causal sequences that link health services to reduced morbidity, mortality, and disability. First, suburban residents, particularly women and children, have better access to and make more use of preventive measures, such as periodic physical examinations, immunization, routine X-rays of the chest, and cytological screening for cancer of the uterus. Such measures definitely reduce morbidity and mortality rates for infectious disease and probably for cancer. Second, prompt, effective treatment of a medical crisis, such as appendicitis, is more readily available to the affluent segment of the community, and surgical complications and death are correspondingly lower. Third, moving childbirth from the home to the hospital, and the development of maternal and infant care programs for previously inadequately served populations have been major factors in the dramatic reduction we have experienced in infant and maternal mortality. Finally, in the areas of mental health and chronic disability, though the extent of illness in different groups is notoriously difficult to measure, it is clear that the well-to-do are more likely to obtain individualized care, whereas the poor are more likely to be neglected or institutionalized. Under these circumstances, "good" care, whether or not it cures the disease, at least helps to prevent the manifestly harmful effects of "bad" or no care.

Historical trends reinforce the idea that purposeful professional intervention contributes to improved health. We have actually overcome much infectious disease. The ideas about how it could be done originated among physicians and others searching for a rational approach to the control of disease. Suppression of many diseases continues to depend upon specific activities of health workers, such as immunization and early detection and treatment, complementing the protection afforded by sewage and water purification systems.

The point is not to deny that general social and economic progress has played an important part in improving health, or to minimize the effect of such extraneous factors as environmental pollution, but rather to reassert the fact that health services, as they have become more rational and scientific, have made a major contribution to the improvement of human health. To suggest that services are "largely unrelated to the health status of the population" is nihilistic and unsupported by the facts. In our zeal to tackle current problems, let us not forget how recently the life of man was short and beset with illness, and let us acknowledge the progress we have made, incomplete and insecure though it may be.

A healthy way of life

The suburbanite benefits from his circumstances, not only directly through the health services he receives, but indirectly as well, since he can afford to cultivate his health. Access to health services implies other social advantages. Good income and education, safer and less crowded living conditions, and adequate nutrition contribute to health in several ways. In the last chapter we noted that poor people, particularly poor children, make relatively few routine or health maintenance visits. Interviews with urban women indicate that good health practices (exercise, good diet, dental hygiene, and the like) are associated with good health and that both are correlated with higher socioeconomic status (income and occupation). Educational and cultural patterns are probably as important as income in producing such differences.[41] An extensive survey of California residents also demonstrates a positive relationship between good health habits and health status, irrespective of income.[42, 43]

Behavior in relation to health care is a learned response. The value of childhood immunization, systematic health surveillance, and routine dental care is not self-evident and needs to be taught. Early recognition of disease and early entry into an adequate diagnostic and treatment program also require basic knowledge of health and disease, plus the ability and the willingness to turn to doctors, hospitals, and other skilled assistance. The well educated can make the system work for them because they know how to use the telephone, make appointments, and obtain transportation, and how to command respect, courtesy, and information.[44]

Socially and economically powerful people tend to live in the suburbs, and they influence the direction of medical research and services. Diseases that afflict the suburban middle class particularly are more likely to lead to effective action than are diseases associated with poverty or with minority status. Coronary disease is well known to threaten middle-aged businessmen, professionals, and politicians, and it follows that an intensive coronary care unit has become a status symbol for community hospitals. When mental retardation occurs in a prominent and powerful family, such as the Kennedys, money, research, and personnel are directed into the field of mental health. Only with the recent economic and political rise of the black constituency has research on the race-associated disease of sickle cell anemia received significant funding.

On the face of it, mortality, morbidity, use of services, and a number of associated advantages indicate that individuals who live in the suburbs and the residential areas of smaller cities have a decided edge on the rest of the population in terms of health. And yet there is widespread and probably increasing dissatisfaction with existing health services among the suburban middle class. Doctors are said to be uninterested, unavailable, and preoccupied with making money. Hospitals are seen as dehumanizing and compartmentalized for the convenience of the providers rather than the consumers. Everything to do with health services costs too much, and people fear a prolonged, disabling illness, which could produce economic disaster.

What are the reasons for this discontent? The economic concerns are real enough, as we saw in the last chapter. But are costs alone sufficient to explain all this criticism of the health care system by those who seem to be benefiting from it? What kind of health care do people who can afford it really want?

EFFECTIVE PERSONAL HEALTH CARE

Public expectations of the health care system, as determined by sociological studies,[44, 45] are clear and consistent enough to define another major social objective. Simply stated, most people want: effective personal health care, provided by competent and interested persons. Physicians themselves also believe that the effective physician is one who is both professionally competent and personally concerned for his patients.[46]

There are two possible explanations, aside from cost, for the present dissatisfaction with health care. The first is that services are perceived by patients as ineffective and impersonal, though they are really not, and the other is that these defects are real. Before dismissing the notion of faulty perception as mere defensiveness on the part of physicians, we will do well to consider some of the difficulties that stand in the way of getting a clear view of how well health services actually operate.

What exactly do we want?

Throughout this book, and particularly in this chapter, there runs a theme of frustration with the present state of health statistics in the United States. In spite of recent major advances, such as the development of a continuing National Health Survey and a periodic National Health Examination, fundamental questions of health policy cannot be thoroughly examined without expensive special studies. The problems of urban health could surely be clarified by a modest increase in our investment in producing and disseminating health statistics.[47] A nation that prides itself on technical know-how ought to be able to furnish health statistics that are accurate, current, uniform, available, and comprehensible to legislators, administrators, and the average person.

In addition, we need to invest some money and some creative imagination in developing and applying new health status indicators. The invention of the gross national product as an indicator of economic status has been one of the most significant developments in the social sciences in recent years. It has proved invaluable to experts, and it has made budgeting, economic change, and international comparisons more comprehensible to the general public. A similarly sensitive and conceptually sound measure of the health of a population could move us ahead toward a more rational health care system. Some interesting work has been done on this problem. Sullivan, at the National Center for Health Statistics, has reviewed the subject and proposed the "expectation of disability-free lifetime" as a measure, based on mortality data combined with information on disability from the National Health Survey.[48] Indices, which include utilization data (visits to physicians, hospitalization, etc.), as well as mortality and morbidity, have also been proposed, and survey questionnaires have been used to define several characteristics of health, including "positive" evidence of health, such as feeling energetic.[49, 50]

Better vital statistics, essential though they are to knowing where we stand, are not sufficient measures of the quality of health care. Most middle-class Americans are more immediately worried about inflation than about their state of health, but the two interests converge when it becomes plain that the most rapidly increasing item in the cost of living index is medical care. How do we know what value we are getting for our money? How can we be sure that new public programs reduce the inequalities of the system and do not exaggerate them? The task of measuring effectiveness and efficiency has not proved easy. Though the cost part of the cost/benefit ratio is evident enough, we have trouble specifying exactly what we want the output of the system to be.

The control of quality in health care, in the past, has depended mainly upon self-regulation by physicians, with only the perfunctory method of licensure and the last resort of prosecution for malpractice to protect the public from extreme forms of abuse. Inadequate though they may seem now, methods of internal control have a long and respected history in medical practice, and new techniques are being developed today. The older, hospital-based traditions include "rounds," in which a group of doctors examine each other's patients; formal consultation, to obtain more expert advice; and clinico-pathological conferences and "tissue committees," in which clinicians test their diagnostic skills against the ultimate criterion of the autopsy or the pathological specimen.

A second general approach to determining the quality of care and relating it to cost has been to audit medical records, using standards set by a consensus of physicians.[51] This process was formalized and put into law in the Medicare requirement that each qualifying hospital appoint a "utilization review" committee of physicians to examine the records of discharged patients and judge whether the admission was medically necessary and the length of stay appropriate.[52] A new law now extends that mechanism by requiring that regional Professional Standards Review Organizations be established, to detect both excessive and insufficient use of physician, hospital, and pharmaceutical service, measured against detailed standards formulated by physicians.[53] Still more recent proposals picture health services being regulated by government-appointed agencies, with representation from consumers, providers, and others, in a manner analogous to the regulation of public utilities.[54]

Thus, we have at hand instruments for applying normative health service standards, that we can use to prevent obvious abuse of the system. Though such audit methods are used only to a limited extent today, as they become linked to governmental payments, they may lead to the regulation of an increasingly costly service industry in the public interest.

And yet, even if the taxpayer could be sure that all the health care his dollar buys met specified standards of competence and effectiveness, he might still be dissatisfied because a well-organized and well-regulated system does not guarantee the kind of personal interest and concern he also wants.

A personal physician

The impersonality of our mass industrial society is particularly distressing to the individual who needs health care. Illness tends to create dependency and a regression toward the feelings of childhood. In sickness, we yearn for an attentive human being who knows and will care for us. It is unrealistic to expect a doctor to be a surrogate mother to all his patients, but it is not out of the question for him to know them as human beings over an extended period of time, to know and care for other members of the family, to respond to their everyday health needs without large omissions, and to serve as a guide in the increasingly forbidding maze of medical specialties.

Significant changes in the organization of health services, particularly at the primary or ambulatory level, are already being undertaken in response to this clearly articulated popular desire for greater numbers of more available personal physicians. A vigorous renaissance of family practice has been gaining ground since 1969, when the field was officially redefined as a "new specialty" with a three-year residency training program, board examinations, and re-examination every six years.[55, 56] The new-style practitioner is intended to be just such a personal physician, prepared for his task by specific training in family dynamics and the understanding and management of common emotional and interpersonal problems. At present, the diminishing numbers of old-style general practitioners are mainly to be found in rural areas and small towns, whereas various combinations of internists, pediatricians, obstetrician-gynecologists, and general surgeons increasingly provide the primary medical care for suburban residents, with multispecialty outpatient departments serving inner city residents. The degree to which the new family practice movement succeeds will probably depend upon whether the comprehensiveness, flexibility, and personal quality of the service furnished by the family practitioner can compete with the more specific skills of a collection of specialists for the trade of a relatively sophisticated suburban clientele.

Family practice is not the only means by which modern medicine might be personalized. Group practice, if it is planned with this personalization as a goal, can relieve the physician of the crushing work load of an open-ended solo practice and give him more time with individual patients, while, at the same time, the patient has the security of knowing that a reliable substitute is always available when his personal physician is not. The combination of group and family practice would go a long way toward meeting the traditional American desire for a personal physician. These two trends, however, have developed separately, and their convergence may be held back by the fact that many older general practitioners are adamant about the virtues of solo practice. An additional factor may be that prepaid group practice is being boosted today because of its economic advantages rather than its potential for a more patient-oriented style of practice. Group practices that are set up with some degree of consumer control should be able to keep these two objectives in better balance.

Another development, which may serve to increase the human quality of health services, is the acceptance of the nurse practitioner or physician's assistant as a true colleague of the primary care physician.[57] A worried mother is likely to get the reassurance and information she needs about her baby in fuller measure from a nurse who has more time to spend with her than from a harassed pediatrician. There are probably limits to how far a physician-substitute can satisfy the desire for psychological support, however, since much of the needed confidence comes from the knowledge—or the belief—that the person rendering care is the most expert available.

Participation

By and large, the health care system works pretty well for the socially dominant members of the community, most of whom live in the suburbs. These people have reasonably good access to modern scientific medicine and to prevention, early detection, and treatment, and their average state of health is distinctly better than that of rural or inner city residents. We catch a glimpse of the elusive objective of optimal physical and mental health in suburbia, but the effort to grasp it firmly continues to be frustrated because we are pushed in different directions by our scientific and humanistic drives. We have built many hospitals, equipped with the latest intensive care and treatment devices, and we have staffed them with a bewildering array of specialists and superspecialists. We have invented a gigantic system of health insurance, which makes it possible for individuals, with the jobs and the money, to use these services, and we are engaged in promising economic and managerial experiments aimed at increasing the efficiency and controlling the costs of the system. We need still better health statistics and more functional organizations, but already the payoff for the suburban middle class is real in such objective terms as reduced morbidity and mortality and lower rates of institutionalization.

Efficient, effective, but impersonal health care might be tolerable, if the latter were its only drawback. But a deeper discontent stems from the patient's feeling that he is excluded from action and decisions that affect his life. Physicians have enjoyed unprecedented social status in the United States and, in recent years, higher income than any other occupational group. It has been easy for them to maintain a professional mystique and to avoid the time-consuming and frustrating business of patient education.

Suburban middle-class patients have acquiesced in this neglect by treating health services as a purchasable commodity for which the consumer has no more direct responsibility than he does for the production of oil. Such an attitude denies the physical and psychological reality that we can never dissociate ourselves from our health. No physician or educational program can prevent smoking or obesity if the will is lacking. Early detection of disease depends largely upon the healthy person's perception of early symptoms. Chronic illness must be lived with. The quality of the doctor-patient relationship can be improved by the active participation of both members in a more fraternal manner than in the past. As we are awakening to a new sense of personal responsibility for the environment, so we are becoming aware that we cannot abuse and neglect our bodies and then expect a hired technician to set them right. Socially and politically, as well as individually, the citizen is beginning to recognize his capacity and his responsibility for achieving a healthier life.

Winds of change are blowing through hospital corridors. Doctors are finding that their suburban middle-class patients have picked up a surprising amount of medical information, some of it folklore or advertising fantasy but much of it sound. More important even than the intelligent questions of informed patients is the growing health consumer movement. Patients' rights are beginning to be codified and made explicit. Laws now require that the patient's "informed consent" be obtained before surgery or before he becomes the subject of an experiment. Rising malpractice claims are calling some careless and incompetent physicians to account and manifest an adversary relationship that is the modern expression of an ancient mistrust of the powerful physician and his mysterious arts. In legislation, in the diminishing political power of the American Medical Association, in the consumer movement, and in other events, signs are visible that the once supreme position of the physician is being challenged. The educated suburban middle class is learning that by economic and political means health services can be made more responsive to the patient's needs and concerns and less exclusively ordered for the convenience of physicians. A political battle has been joined. Its outcome is not yet clear, but it will surely alter the constellation of power in the health care field.

7 WHO'S IN CHARGE?

Any effort to achieve better and more equitable access to health services in the city immediately encounters political obstacles. A surgeon, attempting to organize emergency services in a large city, finds that he must deal with dozens of departments, public and private hospitals, and a chaotic financing system, with no one person in charge to negotiate with. An administrator, given the task of developing a new neighborhood health center in the inner city, encounters resistance on the part of the mayor, councilmen, private physicians, public health officials, and even from the disadvantaged people he intends to serve. A young physician, thoroughly trained as a new-style family practitioner, finds the staffs of some large urban hospitals closed to him and faces severe economic competition with established specialists.

The stakes are large in the highly serious game of urban health. More than three-quarters of the total national expenditure for health services is spent in metropolitan counties. The urban share amounted to at least $72 billion in the fiscal year 1972-1973, or 5.9 percent of the gross national product. The health "industry" is the third largest industry in the country. Non-governmental health services alone employ 3.4 million people.[1] Nearly seven-eighths of physicians are concentrated in metropolitan counties, plus three-quarters or more of nurses and most other autonomous and allied health workers (Table 5.1).

The economic character of health service transactions has been heavily stressed in this country. The basic economic unit has been defined as the "service" (office, clinic, or home visit, hospital day, etc.) and for each service the patient or a "third party" insurer has had to pay a fee. This method of payment tends to channel services toward those who can pay readily and away from the poor who depend upon restricted public financing and from those of marginal income who must choose between health care and basic necessities. A two-class system of paying for care has developed, symbolized in many large urban hospitals by the contrasts between well-appointed private pavilions and crowded staff (formerly "charity") wards. Granting that slow progress is being made toward democratization of hospitals and other services, the stubborn persistence of wide differentials shows that a hierarchical class and economic system still operates.

A more equitable health care system will only come about in this country if it is introduced in a way that takes realistic account of the power structure. There are three major urban-centered groups with strong vested interests in the operation and control of health care: the group that provides it, the group that manages it, and the group that receives it. The problem is basically political, both in the original Greek meaning of the word (*polis,* city) and in its contemporary sense of "competition between competing interest groups or individuals for power and leadership in a government or other group."[2]

Achieving the objectives for urban health, which have been stated in the first six chapters, will depend upon local and national leadership capable of changing the balance of power among the competing factions. This chapter, therefore, will examine who the players are in the game of urban health and what cards they hold, and the next will consider our political values, which constitute the rules of the game. In the final chapter, we will look at the possibility of reinstituting an old, neglected rule, which could alter the game and improve the outcome for all the players.

HEALTH CARE WORKERS

The doctors

Attention focuses at once on the doctors. By virtue of their extensive training and highly specific social function, reinforced in this century by the increasing technicality of medicine and a politically strong professional organization, physicians in the United States have determined much of the form of health services. Their most apparent influence has been highly conservative.

The physician has been accorded much prestige in American life. An important figure as one of the few learned men in the frontier town, his status was raised still further by the institutionalization of medical education after 1900, on the Johns Hopkins model. Strong economic and social interests have led the practitioner of medicine to hold and foster strongly conservative views. The recent migration of physicians with their private patients to the suburbs has tended to shelter them from contact with the health problems of the urban poor. To the busy practitioner in a large suburb or small city, the health care system may seem to be working well enough. Furthermore, the individual physician's occupational tendency to conservatism has been powerfully reinforced by the strong, unilateral political stance of the American Medical Association, which has consistently fought to retain the small-town, nineteenth-century pattern of health care, characterized by independent solo practice, individual doctor-patient relationships, and, above all, fee-for-service payment.[3]

But the medical profession is not so monolithic as either the AMA or its severest critics would have us believe. Even in a medium-sized Canadian city, a sociological study reveals a stratified power structure within the medical profession.[4] In the United States, many individual physicians, academicians, public health officials, and the AMA itself (before 1920) have been leaders in the social reform of health services.[5] The average practicing physician pursues his vocation with a strong sense of professional responsibility toward his individual patient and little time for social issues. But he is also a pragmatist.[6] As the city has grown up around him, he has adjusted his practice to new complexities. The proportion of physicians in specialty practice, for example, has increased from one-sixth to two-thirds in the past 40 years.[7] The rise of specialism has had more to do with making solo practice obsolete than has any political or social change. In order to get care for their patients and to concentrate on their own field, urban physicians have had to develop informal referral networks, facilitated for many years by various forms of associated practice located in typical "medical arts" buildings where laboratory and X-ray services are convenient and expenses may be shared. In 1931, Rorem found 150 "private group practices" in the United States,[8] and the number has grown slowly but steadily since.

Important innovations in health care delivery have been made by physicians. The Group Health Cooperative of Puget Sound, the largest consumer cooperative in the country, developed out of a prepaid clinic started by a physician in Tacoma in 1912.[9]

Academic physicians, ever since the full-time system was established in 1910, have formed a sizable bloc within the profession, with views on health services that are often at variance with those of the AMA. Since academicians have been increasingly paid by full-time salary, their allegiance to the fee system has been weak. Through their professional organization, the Association of American Medical Colleges, they have become politically active, particularly in pressing for federal support of medical education through research and training grants[10] and, more recently, by direct subsidy, a form of governmental intervention that is highly distasteful to practitioners in the AMA.[11] A few prestigious medical schools have also undertaken ambitious new prepaid comprehensive health care programs for urban populations, such as the Harvard Community Health Plan[12] and the program the Johns Hopkins Medical Institutions are sponsoring for residents of the new city of Columbia, Maryland.[13]

Thus, within the medical profession, town and gown differ. Another frequently dissident group within the medical profession is represented by the schools of public health and their graduates.

A striking example of the impact a public health official can have on urban health services was the action of New York City Commissioner of Hospitals, Dr. Ray Trussell, on leave from his position as Dean of Columbia School of Public Health. In 1961, Dr. Trussell established affiliation agreements, supported by tax money, among the ailing municipal hospitals of New York and several strong teaching hospitals and their medical schools. The step did not resolve the very complex health care problems of that city, but it did move the separate worlds of municipal public and "voluntary" hospitals a little closer together.[14] In the Bronx, a hospital administrator with a public health background, Dr. Martin Cherkasky, was largely responsible for the innovative development of one of the few regionally organized health care systems in a major city.[15]

Other health workers

Physicians are a separate interest group and a powerful one at that, since they virtually control licensing and medical education, which regulates the size of an essential manpower pool.[16] Because of this power, some leaders within the profession have expressed the opinion that medical schools and their teaching hospitals have a unique capacity to solve the problems of health care delivery.[17] Doubt, however, is cast upon this proposition by differences of opinion and interest within the profession itself as well as by the existence of other powerful groups with their own ideas about how health services should function.

Some of these groups are also health workers who assist and sometimes compete with the physician as providers of care. Since 1900, physicians have dropped from 35 to 10 percent of total health manpower despite a 2½-fold increase in numbers.[18] These numerous new health practitioners have evolved and are trained in the large urban hospitals, the size of which permits individuals to devote all their time to aspects of patient care that physicians performed hurriedly or not at all in the past. Established, highly trained workers, such as dentists and nurses, are striving for professional status similar to that of physicians, and a certain amount of political energy is being devoted to the struggle over who will regulate and direct nurse practitioners and physicians' assistants.[19]

Today, health workers at all levels constitute 5 percent of the non-agricultural labor force.[18] Old types of allied health workers, such as nurses' aides and orderlies, are beginning to be supplemented and replaced by new types: community health aides, physicians' assistants, and nurse practitioners.[20] These non-physician health workers are concerned with shifting wage scales and developing career patterns, and they are asking for a fairer share of funds which have flowed mainly to physicians in the past. A degree of vertical social mobility is being introduced into what have traditionally been dead-end jobs, and health workers, particularly those who are unskilled and semi-skilled, have begun to organize and form unions.[21] Wages, as a result, have risen from minimal to subsistence, though not yet to levels competitive with wages paid by other industries. The growing cost of labor has been one of the major causes of the rapid inflation of health care costs. Ironically, the increasing number and growing economic attractiveness of health service jobs helps keep the migration of the poor flowing into large cities. Jobs are the magnet, and the health industry offers more jobs every year.

The hospital, a political arena

The interests of doctors, nurses, therapists, practitioners, aides, orderlies, and the rest of the more than 125 distinct types of health worker converge in the modern hospital, which finds its fullest expression and most dynamic development in the large, urban, university-affiliated teaching hospital and its associated services. Not since the active days of medieval cathedral towns have so many people from so many walks of life congregated in one place to carry out one type of work. The medical center is like a miniature city in which hundreds of people work closely with each other, with an over-all common purpose but many different personal goals and much inevitable friction. A sociological study of one large medical center in an eastern city makes clear the fact that conflict of goals and running battles for prestige and dominance among the staff all too often result in neglect of the patients' welfare.[22] Though physicians give their loyalty first to the profession and second to the institution, less highly trained workers are more hospital oriented.[23]

Large numbers of patients are required to support the functions of a fully developed health service center. Still more patients are required to provide the variety of experience essential for the training of a modern specialist. Thus, hospitals have become a big business, absorbing 38 percent of the nation's $94 billion annual health budget.[24]

In the large urban hospitals, practicing physicians, medical school faculties, and a small army of other health care workers are brought into contact, not only with each other, but also with a large number of administrators, government officials, and businessmen trustees, who, in response to runaway health costs and pressures from the public, are beginning to test and to assert their latent powers. It is doubtful that the large urban hospital has ever been the absolute domain of the physician, but with the advent of such control measures as cost accounting, medical audit, and peer review–with more controls to come–it will surely not be so in the future.

HEALTH CARE MANAGERS

Conservative physicians have long mistrusted "third parties" whom they see as intervening between themselves and their patients. This issue, which troubles physicians in the United States far more than in other countries, has been made prominent by the insistence of physicians themselves on an economic definition of health care, according to which the quality of care depends upon the method of payment, with the direct payment of a fee for service as the symbol of a close doctor-patient relationship. The physician who thinks this way necessarily sees himself as an individual, small entrepreneur, in competition with larger health businesses, such as organized groups, and separated from his patients by governmental and other agencies that pay for services.

Particularly in cities, physicians are giving up this unequal struggle. The AMA reported that 86 percent of physicians were in private practice in 1931 and 73 percent in 1950. By 1967, the proportion had dropped to 61 percent, and in that year, since many physicians "in private practice" were also receiving salaries from hospitals, group practices, and other sources, the term was dropped and a new term, "patient care," substituted.[25] This small change in terminology probably reflects a great change of attitude, acknowledging, as it does, that in modern urban health care more than one-half the patient care hours are provided by institution-based physicians, most of whom are salaried.[26]

Hospital managers in the ascendant

The conservative physician is right in suspecting that a great many people besides himself and his patient have an interest in the delivery of health care. Large university medical centers, for example, are big businesses, run with varying degrees of efficiency under the general supervision of trustees, most of whom are businessmen. The Columbia-Presbyterian Medical Center complex in New York City, for example, had assets of $180 million in 1968, and its trustees included the presidents of U.S. Steel and A.T.&T.[27]

Large hospitals possess increasing regulatory as well as economic power. The importance of the hospital as a social institution was affirmed by the Darling decision in the Illinois Supreme Court in 1965. The court observed that accreditation standards, state licensing regulations, and hospital bylaws, "regard it as both desirable and feasible that a hospital assume certain responsibilities in the care of the patient."[28] This decision marks a major shift of responsibility and hence of professional, economic, and political power from the individual physician to the institution.

In hospitals, as in other large industries, a new managerial class has been developing, at first from the "shop" (i.e., physicians), but now more often lay hospital administrators, trained for the task and able, as mediators between the medical staff and the trustees, to exert a great deal of power. This power is not limited to policy decisions within individual hospitals, important though these decisions are, but may extend to the whole community through hospital associations and planning agencies.

The "health care executive" is already influential and has the potential to become an agent for change in urban health. There are now some 8,000 trained hospital administrators in the country. Their functions include the kinds of fiscal, personnel, and organizational responsibilities described in Chapter 5. New patterns, such as those seen in the Kaiser-HMO system, are beginning to be more widely used, and still newer techniques, such as systems analysis, performance evaluation, and fiscal and marketing surveillance, are being adapted from business practice.[29]

With a few notable exceptions, hospital administrators have not so far become visible leaders in changing the health care system, but physicians and boards of trustees are finding them as indispensable and influential as are managers in other businesses.[30] The ascendant managerial technostructure described in industry by Galbraith has its counterpart in the field of health. Power, he says has passed to "the association of men of diverse technical knowledge, experience or other talent which modern industrial technology and planning require."[31]

The importance of the health care administrator will probably continue to be limited if his field of operations remains confined to the hospital at a time when pressures are building to improve primary care, ambulatory services, and preventive medicine and when general alarm over rising costs of hospital care turns public attention to cost and quality control and to alternatives to hospitalization.

One such alternative is "foundations [or corporations] for medical care," defined as "management systems for health-services delivery, set up and run by physicians." This merger of physician and manager interests has spread from its origin in San Joaquin County, California in 1954 to at least 27 states. The potential of such an organization to gain influence and power is indicated by the fact that opposition has developed from insurance and hospital organizations, and some early steps toward merging foundations and hospitals have been taken.[32]

Managers, generally identified as "planners," are also developing new functions and a new range of influence with the evolution of community, regional, and state planning agencies (Chapter 5). Directors of such agencies and their successor programs will operate on a community-wide scale and be answerable to the public interest under federal law, with an increasing degree of authority to coordinate voluntary hospitals and other services with public programs.

Voluntarism waning

Community leaders–mainly businessmen, but also prominent citizens in many walks of life–have had much to do with managing health and welfare affairs in major cities of the United States during the past 50 years as trustees of voluntary philanthropic service organizations and foundations with health-related purposes. Coordinated budgeting of such agencies originated in Cleveland in 1913 and has extended the influence of the "voluntary sector." In the absence of strong governmental health agencies and programs, organized community philanthropy has often stepped in to regulate and plan health services.[33, 34] Generally reflecting a conservative, business-oriented point of view, these voluntary organizations have also provided a forum for religious, social service, and other community groups interested in the delivery of health care. Some large private foundations have financed important experiments and demonstrations in health services, such as the training of new types of non-physician health workers and the development of model prepaid health care programs. The advent of federal financing of health services and community health planning in the past decade, however, has weakened the influence of voluntary health organizations and raised doubts about their future direction.[35, 36]

Medical industries

Two other kinds of industry have a major stake in the health business: drug manufacturers and producers of hospital equipment, supplies, and an expanding range of technical goods used in health services, from disposable gloves to computers. The relationship of these large and profitable business enterprises to the delivery of health care in the city is indirect but not insignificant. The exceptionally high cost of drugs in this country certainly contributes to the medical indigency of the poor and near-poor, and to the painful escalation of total health care costs of which the affluent suburban resident complains.[37, 38] Businesses that produce and promote complex, expensive new devices for diagnosis, treatment, and hospital operation develop their markets in the giant urban medical centers and thus contribute both to the cost of medical care and to the concentration of resources in large hospitals, without reference to whether this is what is most needed by the community as a whole.[39]

Another group of businessmen who are clearly health care managers are the operators and agents of large insurance firms. Private health insurance was a $20.5 billion business and accounted for more than one-quarter of all personal health care expenditures in 1972-1973.[40] Insurance plans vary widely in their benefits. Many insure only hospital services, and this fact has contributed to the higher rates of hospital utilization by suburban residents, who are more likely to own insurance.[41]

The interests of the health insurance industry coincide to a striking degree with the economic interests of the hospitals. By 1966, one-half the income of general hospitals came from insurance. The nonprofit Blue Cross plans have provided a mechanism for the regular increase of hospital rates without direct pressure on the consumer and for the maintenance of a price structure in which certain hospitals are paid much higher rates than others.[42] One reason for these discrepancies is that some of the costs of research and medical education, particularly for residents who are being trained in medical and surgical specialties, have been included in the daily hospital rate.[43, 44] The capacity of Blue Cross to exert some control over prices has not been used. A dramatic reversal of this policy of passing on educational and research costs to the consumer was attempted early in 1971, when the Pennsylvania commissioner of insurance disallowed all such costs as part of Blue Cross contracts. Other states have since followed this lead, though somewhat more cautiously, and private insurance companies have brought antitrust suits against Blue Cross.

A significant turning point in the power of the health insurance industry came with the passage of the 1965 Medicare law. Surprisingly enough, health care insurers offered no opposition and even some support.[45] Commercial and nonprofit carriers were finding the burden of costs of health care for the elderly unmanageable. The segment of the population with the greatest per capita health needs has the least income with which to pay premiums, and rate increases were already encountering public criticism, if not yet effective resistance.

Governmental managers

The shift of an important segment of health care costs from private insurance to the national Social Security program turns the spotlight on another group of health care managers, the bureaucratic administrators whose influence on the delivery of health care in cities and elsewhere throughout the nation is certainly growing. The decade of the 1960's saw a spate of health-related legislation. Some of it, such as the Poverty (OEO) and Model Cities programs, was directed specifically at solving the problems of unequal distribution of such facilities and services as health care in the cities of the United States. These programs initially attempted to introduce federally funded health care activities directly into urban ghettos. Predictably, they met with resistance from city and state governments. Many American cities have weak health departments, but a few city governments have been able to take control of neighborhood health centers and to assert themselves as strong participants in comprehensive health planning programs.[46]

No group connected with health care is more difficult to identify and describe than the one comprising governmental health officials. These officials are unmistakably growing in number, since public expenditure, which accounted for one-seventh of all personal health care expenditures in 1930, now accounts for two-fifths.[47] An estimated 5,000 persons (other than physicians and nurses) were employed in 1969 in federal, state, or local programs as public health administrators, health program analysts, and health program representatives, compared to 17,200 in hospital administration, 16,000 in nursing home administration, and 8,000 in the operation of voluntary health agencies.[48] This is surely an underestimate, since it omits those persons employed in such large governmental agencies actively dealing with health matters as the Social Security Administration and the National Institutes of Health, to name only two. Government health programs include direct services, ranging from large and shockingly bad state mental hospitals to some highly efficient and effective city health clinics, plus a growing and poorly coordinated set of administrative departments, offices, and programs. The authority of public health officials is limited, whether by statute, by budget, or by competition with the private sector. Federal, state, and local health authorities function under a maze of conflicting laws and are largely independent of each other.[49] Impending national health legislation could change this. Bills now before Congress contain administrative provisions, usually negative, in the form of cost and occasionally quality controls. Senator Kennedy's bill, even after modification, proposes what amounts to a full-scale national health administration. The debate, at this point, however, centers on financing, and the essential decision to be made is whether commercial and nonprofit insurers will continue to dominate the field, reinforced by federal law requiring the purchase of insurance by employers. The insurance companies have been strengthened for this battle by being relieved of the burden of paying for the care of old people, but the price was high. The precedent of direct government health financing set by Medicare is likely to be extended in the future, if not immediately.

We frequently hear today the assertion that health care is a right belonging to all citizens. The logical corollary, that it is the responsibility of government to assure that all citizens have access to health care, is not yet widely accepted, but the direction of change seems clear. Administrators of publicly funded health services are the managers most likely to increase in numbers and influence in the next decade.

HEALTH CARE RECIPIENTS

For many years in the United States consumers have banded together to purchase health care. Certain mutual and fraternal organizations were formed specifically for this reason, and many organizations with other primary purposes have included health insurance among their "beneficial" activities.[50]

Labor unions

Labor unions have taken a particular interest in health services, focusing first on the occupational health hazards of large urban industries and, subsequently, on general health care.[51] The International Ladies Garment Workers Union established the first union health center, in New York City, in 1913. Subsequent efforts of labor unions to operate their own health services met with some success in the largest cities and much difficulty elsewhere, most notably, in the struggles of the United Mine Workers to control health services in the towns and cities of the Appalachian coal fields.[52, 53]

During the wage freeze, at the time of World War II, unions introduced health and welfare benefits as a major object of bargaining, and the resulting large health and welfare funds are important resources in the continuing campaign for consumer-oriented health services. The Teamster Center Program, for example, financed a study of health care in New York City in 1964, which gave substance to the suspicion that union members were receiving care of different quality from different sources.[54]

Community participation

New popular forces have been brought to bear on urban health services during the past decade, associated with the civil rights movement and the War on Poverty. Public consciousness of the plight of the urban and rural poor was greatly heightened during the Kennedy administration. The extensive social legislation introduced then and during the Johnson administration has since encountered many bureaucratic, political, and financial obstacles.[55] Comprehensive Health Planning, Regional Medical Centers, and other programs were modified, cut back, or phased out under the conservative policies of the Nixon administration. Nevertheless, these efforts broke new ground, opening up sometimes highly dramatic points of conflict between health professionals and managers on the one hand and community groups and representatives on the other. The laws establishing these programs required community participation, and social action groups found the health care issue a popular rallying point. Moynihan has told the story of the early days of the OEO in a book with the eloquent title, *Maximum Feasible Misunderstanding*;[56] other observers agree that the sudden concentrated drive to achieve community participation through federal legislation essentially failed.[57]

Organized consumers

But the effort was one that dealt with fundamental social issues, which will persist. Pre-existing and new national consumer organizations have developed clearer and more directed policies in support of health care legislation during the 1970's.[58] Poor people and minority groups have glimpsed the possibility of sharing in decisions that affect their lives directly. Middle-class suburbanites, alarmed at the costs and the impersonality of the system, are also beginning to realize that they have a stake and could have a voice in determining its future. Participation can range from powerless "advisory" functions through grievance and ombudsmen procedures to outright political and financial control. Much more experimentation, education of all concerned, and, probably, conflict lie ahead. Such bitter confrontations as the one over Lincoln Hospital and the Gouverneur Health Services Program in New York City suggest that a fundamental dispute, amounting at times to an open struggle for power over health services, is underway. A review of the subject in 1970 pictured many uncertainties ahead but concluded: "What does seem clear, however, is that the scope and amount of community participation will increase and accelerate, no matter what form it may take in our pluralistic society."[59]

This long-range trend has been decidedly slowed during the ensuing years of the Nixon and Ford administrations' policies of fiscal and political conservatism.[60] The role of the private market has been increased, and limited revenue-sharing has resulted in some uneven decentralization of economic power. The voice of the consumer of health services has been muted, but not silenced.

Sustained efforts by organized labor and consumer groups and a vigorous legislative program have so far failed to establish any broad or consistent base of power for the consumer. The balance, as it exists now, and the probable changes in the near future seem more likely to result in a realignment of authority among health professionals and administrators than a strengthening of the position of the consumer. Still, the poor are no longer as effectively excluded from the system as they were ten years ago, and the discontent of the middle classes, who have great potential political power, continues to rise. Cooperative plans, to which we will return in the final chapter, could provide an effective channel for the expression of the strong natural interest of the ordinary citizen in his own health.

A SHIFTING BALANCE OF POWER

In a detailed case study of the economic and political forces behind the health care services of New York City, Ginzberg and his colleagues find that, despite general agreement on the need for improvement, no one group has sufficient power to make any major changes; and their "outstanding finding is the inertia of the system as a whole."[61]

This pessimistic conclusion has much to support it, especially in the uniquely complex and ponderous situation of New York City. But signs of change can be detected in other urban centers, and historical trends suggest that change is more probable than stasis. The balance of power among workers, managers, and the public is distinctly shifting.

"Power," according to Galbraith, "goes to the factor which is hardest to obtain or hardest to replace."[62] Highly trained and relatively scarce, physicians have long dominated the health care field. Today, however, their once unique authority and skills are beginning to be shared and redistributed among other individuals and institutions. After repeated political defeats, the AMA is losing membership and may not be able to change its orientation and image in time to regain its claim to being the voice of the profession. Academic medicine, at the end of 20 years of generous public support of research, now faces demands for the application of research findings and for the training of more primary care physicians in a shorter curriculum. The admission of a broader social spectrum of medical students will alter the orientation of the profession itself and may accelerate the shift toward public and consumer representation. Physicians' assistants and nurse practitioners, though still few in number, are beginning to take over many of the physician's traditional functions and, in some circumstances, may compete with him for status and income in the future.

Managers are clearly gaining importance and power on many fronts, and good, experienced managers are becoming the "factor which is hardest to obtain." Hospital administrators, as we have seen, have already achieved a position of great influence. Some observers of the health care scene predict that the hospital and its management will nearly pre-empt the system. The hospital, it is said, will become a "center of community health services and planning"[63, 64] or the nodal point of a regional health system.[65] The corollary of such a development would be further magnification of the already impressive power of the hospital administrator, to the degree that the term "hospital" would have to be replaced by a broader term, such as "regional health center." There are, however, internal and external resistances to this trend. Trustees of voluntary hospitals are likely to see the enlargement of ambulatory and extramural programs as a financial burden and a dilution of the original function of their institutions. Large, impersonal institutions are viewed with hostility by many in the community, who cannot understand why such mighty organizations cannot provide adequate primary care.[66] The specialized and research-trained medical staff of large teaching hospitals are not oriented to the provision of primary care. Continually rising costs will probably lead to increased regulation of hospitals and thus to a reduction of their autonomy and, possibly, their importance.

Meanwhile, outside the hospital, other managers are also interested in expansion, on a business or governmental base. The potential of medical care "foundations" is being tested. The power of Blue Cross and other health insurers at the national level hangs in the balance of present legislative proposals. If the purchase of health insurance were to be made compulsory, these organizations would take a new lease on life and could be as influential in shaping health services over the next 30 years as they have been in financing the hospital-centered development of the past 30 years. The more likely alternative is that the trend established by Medicare will continue, with national health insurance managed by the Social Security Administration and new federal agencies.

The insurance companies, in that case, would be reduced to the status of agents in a governmentally regulated system.

If the power of private insurers decreases, that of governmental administrators will surely rise. In the consolidation and probable strengthening of the Health Systems Agencies and their closer affiliation with established state health departments can be discerned the shape of a national health care planning and regulatory system through which increasing proportions of public money will flow.

The main arena in which these issues will be contested is Congress, and their present form is that of legislation proposed and backed by shifting lobbies and coalitions. In the absence of any one prepotent interest group, the leverage of social legislation could be great. Distinctly different bills are being promoted by the American Medical Association, the American Hospital Association, insurance companies, and a labor-liberal coalition. Proposals by the Nixon administration were favorable to the business community in general and the insurers in particular, and early indications are that the Ford administration will follow suit. The result will be that, though the probability of a national health insurance program continues to rise, any action by the 94th Congress will tend to be a compromise of limited scope. Major changes in the American system of health care are most likely to occur when the president and Congress work together. The 1976 election, therefore, may offer the people a new opportunity to install an administration committed to improved health services and able to collaborate with Congressional leaders to that end, as President Johnson did in the case of Medicare.

8 CONSERVATIVES, TECHNOLOGISTS, AND REFORMERS

Since health is a social good, the means taken to achieve it are a public concern, and decisions about which means to adopt are arrived at by a political process. The problems of urban health may be approached from widely different points of view, leading to equally different social actions. This chapter will therefore examine competing versions of the rules of the game.

Four schools of thought on how to deal with the health problems of our cities can be recognized. Conservatives, who have often dominated American public policy in the field of health in the past 50 years, point with pride to the solid achievements of American medicine and assure us that no change in goals will be necessary to guarantee further progress.

Moderates, in contrast, recognize an urgent need for change but propose two different kinds of solutions. One group looks upon environmental pollution and the disorderly state of the health care system as essentially technological problems to be solved by applied science, more research, and better management. The other group defines the problems of civic health as essentially social in origin and proposes that enlightened reform, mainly through federal legislation, will lead to improved health and welfare.

Radicals, however, deny that any technical or social reform can possibly level the economic inequalities and prevent the exploitation of people and natural resources that characterize our present system. Accordingly, we must relinquish customary goals of profits and production in order to improve health, welfare, and social justice.

Each of these four political schools has its ethics, its rationale, and its supporters. None can be disregarded in a pluralistic society, but none offers a complete and fully satisfactory program for improved urban health. We will consider the first three possibilities in the present chapter. In the final chapter we will examine the radical program and then, returning to the neglected democratic principle of fraternity, will suggest how a missing dimension can be restored.

Meanwhile, repeated proclamations of a health care "crisis" suggest that a major battle is about to be joined, and the skirmishes have become more frequent. Since hopes for better urban health hinge on the outcome of this battle, let us examine what ground each party holds and what action it calls for.

THE CONSERVATIVE VIEW

The official view held by the organized medical profession has long been that the United States has the best health care in the world and that the existing system will continue to function well as long as it is not interfered with by government, or other "third parties."[1] Practicing physicians have generally been supported in this attitude by political conservatives, who have admired the solo, fee-for-service practitioner as the last stronghold of individual enterprise. The conservative camp has had a more uneasy alliance with other vested interests in the health field, such as those of the hospitals and insurance companies, which cannot adopt exactly the same position since they cannot insulate themselves entirely from the needs and pressures of the larger community.

Since the conservative plan for the future is basically one of no change, no new proposals are offered. The campaign is based, instead, on calling attention to past and present achievements.

Indeed, there is much to be proud of in the record of American medicine. In our large urban hospitals and teaching centers, we have assembled research and specialized diagnostic and treatment facilities of high quality, and these resources form an essential base for future development. Even in the absence of a national health policy, we have managed to direct a higher proportion of our national resources to health services and research than has any other large developed country. Medical schools attract more of our academically best qualified students than can be accommodated, and the training of non-physician health workers has expanded even more rapidly than the population. As measured by such indices as maternal and infant mortality, we have recently fallen behind comparable countries, but this fact cannot obscure the great and sustained progress we have made over the past century in controlling epidemic infectious disease, in making childbirth and infancy safer, and in protecting the working man from injury. Bad though health conditions may be in our inner cities, they are better than on the small farms of poor rural areas, and they are better largely because the city does have more and better services. Finally, conservatives would stress that the value of individual freedom–professional freedom for the physician and "freedom of choice" for the patient–has been staunchly defended in the field of medicine.

Can this list of accomplishments justify the conservative attitude that evolution will bring still more improvement if we will just refrain from tinkering? Aware of the conditions of health in large segments of our population, only a citizen with an overriding puritanical faith in the moral necessity of poverty and suffering could agree. The gains have been made at a high cost. By treating health care strictly as a salable commodity, we have bought good care for many citizens but denied it to the poor. No system of dole has yet been devised which can abolish the inequalities of personal and public health care between the inner city poor and those who can afford and know how to use the system.

Marginally profitable or commercially uninsurable health services, such as those offered by nursing homes and mental hospitals, are inadequate, inferior, or both, and occasional examples of outright exploitation make the picture bleaker still. Primary care has simply been disappearing from our inner cities, and no government or agency can be held responsible. Voluntary hospitals are being overloaded by demands for ambulatory and emergency care the hard-pressed city governments and limited private endowments cannot finance. Over the whole city hangs the pall of automotive and industrial waste, which is taking its toll of health and life and which we will certainly not be able to eliminate by simply letting things drift. Change is imperative. Can it be made without sacrificing the incentive, the flexibility, and the power of the money-based system that has brought us where we are?

TECHNOLOGICAL PROGRESS

Moving left from extreme conservatism, we encounter a more popular but still essentially elite viewpoint: that of business, engineering, or science. Though they work in different contexts, individuals in these three fields tend to approach health care similarly. They take a pragmatic view, analyzing problems of urban health as a malfunctioning machine that needs adjustment and new inputs and feedback controls. If the desired output can be specified in quantitative terms and if available resources and unwanted side effects can be identified, then the system can be redesigned or programmed accordingly. Historically, this viewpoint has been gaining ground steadily since the beginning of the Industrial Revolution, and it is powerfully supported by the fact that it has essentially created the man-made world in which we live.

Managerial ideology

Closely associated with the scientific and engineering viewpoint is that of business, in which new technology is adapted and, at least in theory, similar scientific and rational principles are used in the management of production processes. "Health care," says

Kerr White, "is a service industry with socially determined ends."[2] Though it is questionable whether society in general is really able to determine ends when they conflict with goals set by a professional and managerial elite, there is little doubt about the fact that business values and practices are being consciously introduced into health care. Conventional wisdom among decision-makers in both Britain and America holds that a health care system, whether a hospital, a regional system, or a prepaid group, should be run like a business.[3]

Managerial thinking seems progressive, in contrast with the laissez faire that has characterized American hospitals in the past, and it has been readily adopted in such newer organizations as the national social action programs of the 1960's and the resulting "health maintenance organizations." As Krause points out, however, this "managerial ideology" serves to align such programs with the dominant technocratic power structure; thus, it is helping preserve the status quo rather than leading to change.[4]

Centralization of planning and administration is a key managerial principle. In one of the few studies relating organizational structure to performance, Roemer and Friedman made a detailed comparison of California hospitals that differed from each other in the degree of discipline of the medical staff. They found that a higher degree of discipline promotes technical excellence and, in turn, improves the standing of the hospital in a wide range of inpatient and community responsibilities. Confirming the present analysis, they reported a marked degree of conflict between individualistic and organizational values in hospitals in the middle range in terms of discipline. In considering future trends, they advocate an organizational pattern that is relatively highly disciplined (full-time department heads) but that retains important functional relationships with professional activities outside the hospital (strong attending staff, rather than all full-time physicians).[5] A step toward uniform regulation of the practice of medicine was taken with the passage of the Professional Standards Review Organization (PSRO) law (PL 92-603), which offered physicians a grace period during which they could establish their own regionalized quality control apparatus in lieu of direct governmental regulation. In spite of initial resistance, it appears that physicians are beginning to accept the inevitability of such a logical administrative development.[6]

Another central idea in modern business practice is regulation of the flow of information. Automation and systems analysis can produce an improved informational data base, which is the major input of the health care system. Record linkage is proposed to bring together the fragmentary and encapsulated bits of personal medical histories a mobile population scatters among hospitals, clinics, and doctors' offices.[7] The hospital medical chart can be converted from a historical document into a flexible instrument for decision-making, coordination, and quality control.[8] The potential value of an improved system of collecting and disseminating national health statistics was noted in the previous chapter. Computer technology offers other improvements in health care. It can aid the physician in collating information and in making a diagnosis. Already, it facilitates appointment systems and financial operations in large hospitals and clinics. An even more promising possibility is that, by means of terminals designed for use by patients, it could enable the patient to gain better access to the system and even to participate more actively in decisions about treatment.

Still another basic principle of management, one that is beginning to be called into question in the industrial world just as it is gaining ground in the health care industry, is that of continual growth, justified by presumed increases in efficiency and "economies of scale." The problem of the scale of health services is a critical one, to which we will return in the next chapter.

Research-mindedness

Modern American industry has been built on a strong faith in the manageability of the world around us. Medical and health care research are also based on a belief in the capacity of the human mind to understand how systems work and to manipulate them for rational purposes. Brilliant successes have resulted from medical research as typified by the reductionistic pursuit of the causative agents of bacterial disease. Most modern investigators of cancer and heart disease use a conceptually similar though more complex model of multiple causes. Research on the "urban factor" in these diseases, which was reviewed in Chapter 1, is motivated by the expectation that once the mechanism of disease causation is adequately understood, control or preventive measures can be applied at the most vulnerable point in the system.

The information required for scientific and technological progress and the transactions by which that progress is achieved are concentrated in large urban universities and research institutes. An early benefit to the health of city dwellers is promised by the control of pollution caused by industrial production, heating, and transportation. London and New York, for instance, have both been able already to establish some control over smoke by regulating the type of fuel burned, and the means for reducing industrial and automotive effluents are undergoing rapid development. Another urgent technological problem related to health is that of developing a mass transport system to compete successfully with the flexibility and convenience of the private automobile.

Additional promising technological progress lies immediately ahead. White has proposed a list of areas that are ready for development, including automated laboratories and record systems, organized and effective emergency services, and restorative aids and devices for the disabled.[2] Probable, but more speculative, are such innovations as the adaptation of aerospace technology to health services.[9] Recent developments in cancer research suggest that the next major advance in scientific understanding may come in this field.

The program of research and development has been demonstrated to be workable, and most Americans are prepared to believe that technology, which has progressively relieved them of so many of the ancient burdens of manual labor and housekeeping, can also protect them from disease and suffering. How, then, is it possible that we still have an almost totally uncoordinated system of health care with large gaps and inefficiencies and that there is as yet no recognizable public mandate to technology to get on with the job?

Limits to technological progress

A reason frequently given is that doctors have resisted change. Certainly the conservative element of the medical profession has slowed progress, particularly progress toward more efficient organization. But the political power of the medical profession has probably been exaggerated in the past and is now distinctly diminishing. Furthermore, most modern physicians are as ready to accept practical changes as are most other Americans. There are other explanations.

Growth and profit, which are the standard criteria for success in business, are not sufficient criteria for the evaluation of health services. To be sure, there is considerable financial profit to be made in such situations as specialty practice or proprietary hospitals, where the providers can select and shape the market. Well-managed health industries, such as certain large private clinics and prepaid plans, have shown remarkable growth. But when the cost of providing services to large segments of the population who are heavy users and not self-supporting (the aged, the disabled, the mentally ill) are averaged in, the total financial cost of health care clearly exceeds any directly realizable income. A more accurate balance sheet, which would take into account such long range social gains as extended life, better health, more productivity, and improved quality of life, still remains to be invented. Even if it existed, it would be extremely difficult for modern managers to assign priorities to alternative outputs, such as longer life for stroke victims, more complete immunization for school children, decreased incidence of lung cancer, or reduced costs. As we begin to formulate these choices in order to develop national policy, it becomes increasingly clear that science and technology alone cannot be relied upon as guides.

Moreover, science and technology are meeting with unaccustomed public resistance because of the undesirable, dangerous, and possibly cataclysmic side effects of some research and development, which has been applied too hurriedly. The public and the Congress are beginning to question whether we must build larger and faster planes simply because we know how to do so or whether we must stockpile more nuclear weapons when we already have enough to destroy any potential enemy many times over. Industrial waste, which seemed harmless when we thought the continent was inexhaustible, is now being recognized as a danger to our health.

Technological backlash is occurring in medicine as well, as toxic side effects of potent drugs, unnecessary surgery, and errors in medical judgment are becoming more widely known to the popular press, public agencies, and the courts.

The opinion is probably more widely held today than ever before that the objectives of business, and even science, useful though they are, are not sufficient to meet the needs of a modern urban society. Somehow, we must define our social goals more thoroughly and organize ourselves better to achieve them. Increased production, energy consumption, and acquisition of new knowledge may all be essential to the achievement of better urban health, but they need direction and social control if they are to serve all citizens.

SOCIAL REFORM

A broad constituency

Advocates of social reform view the health care problems of urban Americans as the result of economic inequalities produced by regional and historical social trends. Poor people, for example, who migrate to cities seeking economic opportunities, are trapped in poverty by outmoded social institutions and the automation of industry. Reformers see the "community of solution" as including at least an entire metropolitan region and sometimes overlapping state boundaries. Such broad definitions lead naturally to efforts to solve health problems by new legislation, sometimes in a single state, but more often at the national level. New laws are implemented by the power of taxation to redistribute resources among the uneven levels of our society. Technical means, particularly those of business management, may also be used to achieve social reform. A potential conflict exists, however, between the goals of efficiency and those of human welfare, and this conflict is increasingly evident today.

A broad constituency, including some physicians, has supported moderate social reform. In an incisive study of the American Medical Association, Richard Harris pointed out that many physicians favored some form of social health insurance before the AMA launched its major campaign of opposition in the 1930's —and many still do.[1]

The bulk of the political support for reform, however, has come from labor. The coalition of southern Democrats and urban workers President Roosevelt put together lasted for at least 35 years. President Johnson's War on Poverty, with its emphasis on urban health problems, was really an extension of the New Deal. As de Toqueville foresaw, egalitarian progress has led to "administrative despotism" and an enormous federal bureaucracy.[10] Since many federal administrators are charged with carrying out the programs of social change Congress has enacted, they, too, may usually be counted among the supporters of this political approach. Leadership and influential support have also been drawn from the professions, particularly education, and from liberal and reform-minded people in every walk of life.[11]

Urban health programs

The agony of our cities has given rise to many efforts to bring about social change. Welfare reform, guaranteed annual income, educational reform and desegregation, the salvaging of disastrous "urban renewal" projects, and the political regeneration of the city on a metropolitan or even megalopolitan scale are examples, and all of them will affect the health of the city dweller. Surprisingly little attention, however, has been paid to health factors in city planning as it is now practiced.[12] For this reason, it will be more instructive to examine some proposals and experiments that concern health care specifically and to question how they relate to other trends of the urban future, rather than speculate on the reverse relationship.

Proposals for the reform of health care in the cities of the United States have been closely tied to efforts to eliminate poverty and racial discrimination. A good example is the program drawn up by a committee assembled by the Department of Health, Education and Welfare in 1967. Their report was entitled *Delivery of Health Services for the Poor*.[13] It made explicit the rationale for health care innovations included in the War on Poverty. "There is an undisputable association," the report stated, "of increased morbidity and mortality with poverty." Though these educators, public health officials, and government administrators made a few technical suggestions, such as the use of helicopters to reach rural areas, the substance of their plan was social reform. Specific goals were "to reduce social and cultural barriers," to assure "more accessible ambulatory care" and "interaction of the health care system . . . with education, welfare, employment, recreation, and corrections," and above all, "to eliminate the financial barrier to the receipt of comprehensive health services for all medically needy (by 1975)." In comparison with these high aims, the measures proposed, such as improved outpatient services and training of ancillary personnel, seem modest, but they were based on careful calculation of how far social reform might practically be pressed under the existing circumstances, which included an escalating war. Some of the specific steps recommended in this report have in fact been tried. Though they have fared unevenly under the continued pressure of the war and the succeeding conservative administrations, they were imaginative social experiments that we must examine critically for what they imply for future developments in health care.

Some of the most important experiments of the last decade have centered on ambulatory health services. These include community mental health centers, children and youth and maternal and infant care programs, and neighborhood health centers initiated by a federal agency, the Office of Economic Opportunity (OEO). Because they were boldly conceived, the neighborhood health centers offer a particularly instructive example of the potential, and also some of the difficulties of social reform in the field of health.

Neighborhood health centers

Under the authority of the OEO (1964), 150 neighborhood health centers were established for the benefit of the medically indigent, mainly in the slums of large cities, but with a few in rural areas.[14]

The idea of a neighborhood health center is not new. The lineage of the present centers extends back to another era of progressive reform in the early years of this century.[15] In several major cities, health stations were established at that time, embodying the principles of outreach (district location), community participation, and bureaucratic organization and centralization of community health and social services. These centers were based on a "social gospel" of service to the poor. Because of the strength of the medical profession at the time, they did not venture into diagnosis and treatment but concentrated instead on such public health activities as improving infant nutrition and providing an immunization program. Between the two world wars the movement lapsed, only to be revived in its present form.

The centers have several purposes and have taken different forms in each community, under the guidance of local trustees. They all share at least three general goals: to attack poverty and discrimination, to bring services where they are needed, and to improve organization and coordination of services. Some of the means adopted to achieve these goals are essentially managerial, such as cost accounting, centralized financing, medical audit, and uniform record keeping. Technological and business methods, as we have noted, can be useful means of achieving reform. But it is striking that at present the entire neighborhood center program is under attack, on the basis of excessive costs and impracticality. Social and technological progress, evidently, are unevenly yoked, if not at times pulling in opposite directions.

The importance of the neighborhood centers lies in their social innovation. A particularly daring move was the requirement, written into the law, that "consumers" would constitute a majority on the boards of trustees charged with management of the centers. Flying in the face of the physician's traditional autonomy and disregarding the existing hierarchy of state and city health services, this political venture stirred up vigorous and sometimes damaging conflict, which is far from being resolved.[16] Whatever their ultimate fate, the centers have confronted a number of urban communities with the reality that patients in general and poor patients in particular have in the past had very little to say about what sort of health services they need and want.[17] Future planners will have to take into account the now established fact that consumer participation is possible and that it leads to a different end result than planning and control from the top down exclusively.

Another important innovation attempted by the neighborhood

health centers has been to use the developing health services as a means of attacking poverty and racial discrimination. Several methods have been adopted, such as placing the centers in areas of greatest need, seating local representatives on the boards, and recruiting staff members from the immediate neighborhood to be served. These health aides have functioned to break down barriers between professionals and medically inexperienced and mistrustful patients. In return, the new workers have been given jobs and on-the-job training to equip them for advancing careers in the health field. Thus, the centers become directly linked with more extensive efforts to solve the underlying problems of urban poverty. It makes sense for urban in-migrants seeking jobs to find them in expanding health services and for a health center to concern itself with the social welfare of its own staff.

Here again, reform encounters resistance. Untrained and poorly educated aides are inefficient, established health workers dislike competition, and the pattern of dead-end jobs at the bottom of the health service pyramid is difficult to change. The centers, initially set up to serve only poor people, have had difficulty developing a clearly defined and active constituency. They have also generally lacked a clear functional relationship to hospitals, with the result that community orientation is lost at a critical juncture in health care.

Despite these obstacles, the centers have already demonstrated that health services can function intimately with their communities without sacrificing quality. Proof of this has been furnished by a study in which a sample of 35 neighborhood health centers was evaluated and compared with other providers of health care by means of medical record audit.[18, 19] The quality of care furnished by the centers was rated slightly above that offered by medical school-affiliated hospital outpatient departments in medicine and pediatrics and slightly below in obstetrics.

A great weakness of the neighborhood health centers is their financing. Being dependent on Congressional appropriations, the very objectives of the program are subject to annual political pressure, change, and even sudden death. Efforts to strengthen the financial base of comprehensive services to a poor population by tapping all potential sources of federal, state, and local support plunge the program planners into a maze of overlapping, inconsistent, and conflicting laws, regulations, guidelines, and arbitrary restrictions that inflate the cost of services and cool the ardor of the most enthusiastic reformer.[20] These are soluble problems, however, which can be dealt with by a strong administration.[21]

A more serious fault in the funding of the centers from the viewpoint of social reformers is that they are special programs designed for poor people. As such, they presuppose the existence of fixed social differences and actually reinforce a class-related system of health care. By providing free care for those who can qualify as sufficiently poor, as Fein points out, the centers restrict the recipients' freedom to select what they consider to be the best health care.[22] Special funding also forces the centers to compete for support with other programs that are attempting to deal with related social problems, instead of with other health care providers with whom they must ultimately compete economically. The obvious way out of the dilemma is national health insurance, which would give all citizens the means to choose their health care–a choice which at present is largely restricted to those who have enough income and insurance to meet rising health costs.

National health insurance

This country has been moving unsteadily toward national health insurance for half a century, and it now seems to be close to enactment. The implications of this reform extend well beyond financial matters, and the way the law will be written could either advance or slow social progress.

National health insurance will be most likely to improve access and maximize equality if it provides universal coverage and comprehensive benefits, and if it is administered by a socially responsible agency, such as the Social Security Administration, as independent as possible of changing administrations.

The first benefit to flow from such a program would be to free the poor from the restrictions of medical indigency and the indignities of welfare investigation. As we have learned from the painful lesson of Medicare, however, financing alone does not create new services. Instead, by putting pressure on limited resources, it inflates costs. Medical insurance, therefore, should logically implement a national policy and become part of a national health system, accompanied by incentives for the expansion, redistribution, and increased efficiency of all health services, from private offices through the largest teaching hospitals.

The most serious deficiency in American urban health services is the inadequacy of primary health care in areas of concentrated poverty. The underlying reason for this maldistribution is that there is no effective way to meet the costs of everyday health service for people who can neither pay the going rates for office visits nor afford insurance against hospital expenses. If every citizen had a legally established right to receive the health service he needed, plus the means to obtain it, we could apply many of the social innovations that have already been shown to be workable.

Our experiences with neighborhood health centers have shown that competent physicians can be attracted to the inner cities, given satisfactory working conditions and adequate salaries. Models for the organization and delivery of comprehensive care are being developed by some leading medical schools in order to prepare their students for imminent changes in professional practice. These experiments are proving to be costly and almost prohibitively complicated to get started because there is at present no reliable way of meeting costs. If it were not necessary to develop and market health insurance programs, these and other important experiments in health care delivery could serve many more patients and get on with the vital business of health care itself. Once financing is secure, the experimenters could concentrate on such problems as redistributing the work of health care so that the most highly trained do the most complex tasks, developing effective methods of teamwork and information exchange, reaching those unable to come to health centers, and effecting the participation of health care recipients in decisions that influence their own lives.

In addition to improvements in personal health services, centralization of health care financing would make possible the systematic allocation of funds to manpower training, the development of new facilities, and the provision of public health services.

The latter has been shown in international studies to be the one variable in health care financing that correlates with reduction in infant mortality.[23]

Other reforms

The device of federal matching funds has been shown to be of limited usefulness in strengthening local health services without abrogating local initiative and private philanthropy. The Hill-Burton Act (1946), intended primarily to encourage the building of small hospitals outside urban areas, has been very successful in effecting exactly that. Many small communities now have excellent facilities, though physicians may be lacking to staff them. Matching fund programs, however, being categorical, tend to develop parts of the system lopsidedly. The early experience of the State of New York with the funding of Medicaid is a case in point. New York established such liberal criteria for eligibility that the need for matching funds nearly bankrupted the state and forced cutbacks in other services. Other legislative devices are also available, such as tax incentives to encourage the development of group practices and neighborhood health centers in the urban and rural areas now being deserted by physicians. Modest federal and state programs aimed at attracting medical students and physicians to underserved areas have shown some encouraging but uneven results.

Social reform can also be achieved by repealing outdated laws. In New York City, during the first year after the adoption of the most liberal abortion law in the country, the abortion rate approached the live birth rate, the maternal mortality rate dropped to less than one-half that of the previous year, and public health officials were expressing surprise at how "smoothly, efficiently, safely and inexpensively it's all worked out."[24] The apparent success of this bold experiment, the repeal of laws based on ancient religious and social attitudes, demonstrates that social reform can have direct effects on health. In her book, *The Economy of Cities,* Jane Jacobs suggested that economic innovation often, if not always, originates in cities and then spreads to towns and rural areas.[25] In the experience with legalization of abortion, we have evidence that health care innovation is also likely to occur first in cities. Though the initiating event was a new state law, in fact, the political action originated in New York City and 80 percent of the abortions in the state during the first year were performed there.

Increasing social tolerance of previously ostracized behavior, such as abortion, illegitimate birth, and homosexuality, will profoundly affect the conditions of health in the city, and legislative changes both reflect and facilitate this tolerance.

Men and women have often been fascinated by the idea of starting a new, healthier, and more rationally organized community. Modern ideas about planning new towns were first put forth in the 1898 Garden Cities proposals of Ebenezer Howard.[26] Though the many new towns and new cities that have since come into being offer an obvious chance to reorganize health services as well as transportation, housing, and other urban functions, it is only very recently that this opportunity has been seized. A new health care system in the new city of Columbia, Maryland, is under development by the Johns Hopkins Medical Institutions and the Connecticut General Life Insurance Company, through the agency of a separate corporation, set up for the purpose of planning a prepaid, voluntary health insurance plan open to all citizens of Columbia.[27]

A physical break-up and reorganization of large cities can be observed, as population shifts from central cities to the suburbs and new clusters form around shopping centers or former towns now incorporated in the metropolis. The development of larger and stronger units of metropolitan government, as in Toronto,[28] is evidence that the simple pattern of central city and politically independent suburbs is already outdated. The megalopolis is here, and the realities of governmental organization are slowly catching up. The change is great and surely significant for health.

Social reform of health care, thus, is popular and in line with both historical tradition and certain recent political trends. Reform to date has repeatedly been shown to be practical and effective, and there are unmistakable signs that more change is urgently needed. Why then, do we continue to put up with intolerable health conditions and fragmented services and to palaver endlessly over such urgent measures as national health insurance?

Limits to social reform

Opposition to social reform is probably more substantial and more deeply seated than is opposition to technological progress. In addition to categorical rejection by conservatives, moderate reformers have to face more cogent criticism by practical scientists and businessmen who point out weaknesses in massive social programs, such as self-defeating bureaucratic complexity, lower priorities for basic research, and the impracticality of open-ended social commitments. Especially, social reform threatens to cost too much. Aside from extravagance, graft, and waste, which are not unique to the operation of social programs, the problem of how much we can afford to spend on health is a fundamental question of national priorities. Since we have been increasing such expenditures rapidly and steadily since World War II, objections to costs do not appear to be based on any necessary limit, but rather on a priority system. Recent history indicates that health care is a rising priority for the American public. Costs, like other potential conflicts between technological progress and social reform, are probably negotiable and manageable. A coalition of the two moderate groups could surely command majority support and bring about changes in our health care system that are both practical and humanitarian. Why doesn't it happen?

Several social critics have diagnosed a recent malaise the citizens of this country seem unable to shake off. "Failure of will" it might be called. Even in the midst of proposing more reform, we are stricken with doubt. Will the price of a national health service be dehumanization of care? Can we control costs and regulate quality without killing initiative and motivation? Can any moderate and progressive action prove adequate to cope with the massive social and technological changes that we face? Self-doubt, even among the most energetic proponents of reform, seems to lie close to the surface and to be a major hindrance to progress in health care.

9 HUMANIZING URBAN HEALTH

The sense that life in American cities is being bled of its humanity is strong. In previous chapters we have observed that urban man can be alienated from himself and from his fellows by mindless industrial work, by the cruelty of city streets, by poverty, by the loneliness of old age, and, above all, by a sense of helplessness in attempting to deal with strong vested interests and with increasingly big, impersonal institutions.

The question raised in this final chapter is whether we can overcome our doubts, reshape our personal lives and institutions on a human scale, and restore to them the strength that arises from close, dependable interaction among human beings who care about each other. Specifically, can we achieve the objective of human relationships within small groups of health workers and recipients characterized by affection and shared values and goals?

RADICAL CHANGE

The gap between this objective and the reality of fragmented services, crowded clinics, and destructively rising costs is great enough to generate anger and a call for radical change. The examples of China and Cuba show that, in two very different social and political situations, great improvement in the health of an entire nation can be achieved by revolutionary efforts.

China and Cuba

In China, the progress in public health and social welfare achieved during the past 20 years has impressed Western observers.[1, 2, 3] Though definitive demographic and epidemiological data are lacking, the available evidence support claims that in the People's Republic of China the lives of one-fifth of the world's population have been radically changed for the better in the past 20 years.[4] One of the poorest of nations, by means of concerted social action, has been able to put into practice the precepts "put prevention first," "in medical and health work, put the stress on the rural areas," and the national motto, "serve the people."

Effective birth control and family planning is said to have halved the birth rate in China. Mortality, particularly among infants, has probably been reduced by more than 100 percent since the establishment of the People's Republic in 1949. Virtual eradication of such historical plagues are cholera, smallpox, malaria, and even venereal disease has been achieved in less than one-half the years required for similar progress in Western countries. Malnutrition has been virtually wiped out. The principal means employed have been the direct application of basic principles of public health and hygiene, through decentralized medical services with simply trained "barefoot doctors" supported by mobile medical teams, rotation of urban physicians into rural areas, and, most important, the mobilization of the public to eliminate disease-carrying pests, to construct hygienic waste-disposal systems, and to coordinate nutrition, maternal care, immunization, and other public health measures. The *Peasant Village Physician's Handbook* presents the principles and practical measures of both Western and traditional medicine in simple language for the guidance of health workers throughout China.[5]

Another glimpse into the possibility of a radically different future is afforded by the experience of Cuba. In 1953, Castro identified health as one of the six major problems he intended to tackle, the others being land-use, industrialization, housing, unemployment, and education. By 1968, despite the flight of one-third of its physicians, Cuba had expanded medical education to the point where there were 1,000 more physicians than before the Revolution. The health budget had increased eightfold, and dramatic improvement had been achieved in infant and maternal mortality rates and in death rates from poliomyelitis, malaria, and typhoid.[6]

This progress has been confirmed by an American public health expert who worked in Cuba in 1972.[7] He reports that under a national policy that attaches high priority to health care, with emphasis on prevention, scarce resources have been centralized, whereas ambulatory care has been decentralized in local health centers. As in China, established measures of public hygiene have been widely applied by the coordinated efforts of all types of people, and large numbers of new workers have been introduced into the health care system, particularly at the less highly trained levels of nurses, nurse assistants, and auxiliary personnel. The contrast with the lack of change over the same two decades in the comparable situation of the Philippines strikingly demonstrates how much has been accomplished in Cuba.[8]

These impressive achievements in China and Cuba offer lessons and inspiration to other developing countries. They may also have significance for industrialized countries, such as the United States, despite profound social and historical differences. Bold social experiments, conducted with what many considered to be prohibitively inadequate resources, have produced remarkable effects. Redistribution and equalization of resources and access have been accomplished to a substantial degree, and the value of centralized planning, high national priority for health programs, and decentralized authority for local services has been demonstrated.

The experiences of China and Cuba are particularly relevant to the theme of this chapter because of the effective way in which the thought, interest, and efforts of average citizens have been mobilized for the promotion of personal and public health. Recent observers returning from China stress the active involvement of the whole population in practical matters of health and hygiene. The phenomenon is clearly political, in that it stems from broad national health "laws," which are systematically indoctrinated, but the intensive efforts put forth by workers at all levels, during "non-working" hours, testify to the fact that the communal striving for better health is part of a deeply felt common social experience. The Chinese phrase "walking on two legs" means not, as the Westerner might think, acting with personal independence, but rather mass involvement of the people combined with skillful guidance by trained professionals.[9]

American radicalism

In the United States, the radical view of urban health begins with an angry denunciation of the inhumanity of our present system. The main target is the "medical-industrial complex," which is not an imaginary scapegoat, as the analysis of the medical power structure in Chapter 7 indicates. The Medical Committee for Human Rights, organized in 1964, and The Health Policy Advisory Center, formed in 1968 in New York City, recently formulated the need for radical change in American health care.[10] The title of a book published in 1970 by Health-PAC identified the enemy as *The American Health Empire: Power, Profits, and Politics:* "The crisis experienced by the poor and middle-class consumer of health care can be traced directly to the fact that patient care is not the only, or even the primary, aim of the medical care system. . . . The demand is to turn the medical system upside down, putting human care on top, placing research and education at its service, and putting profit-making aside."[11]

Current sociological views of the health care system have been summarized by Waitzkin and Waterman, who also present their own radical critique in *The Exploitation of Illness in Capitalist Society.*[12] In addition to the imperialistic character and social stratification they find to be associated with medicine, they point out that the "sick role" can provide a retreat for oppressed individuals and can be used by dominant providers, along with control of medical information, to blunt protest and maintain the status quo.

Some radical thinkers like Ivan Illich go still farther and classify the health care system along with education as an institution that has lost its socially constructive purpose and become in itself a source of illness and ignorance.[13]

Outspoken advocates of radical change in the health care system are not numerous, but they are being listened to attentively by many young people, among them students in the health professions and such allied fields as social work. Radicalized youth, militant blacks, underpaid health workers, and many whose work brings them into close contact with the poor, point to public hospitals, with their crowded "staff" (formerly "charity") wards and bleak outpatient clinics, as part of a social pattern, which, in effect, excludes the poor from everyone else's life. Causes for protest are abundant, and the limited successes of such measures as the neighborhood clinics throw into relief the great unmet need. A trip through the average state mental institution is enough to make the most conservative citizen think, at least for a moment, that something drastic must be done. What are the radical proposals?

No single program has yet evolved, but certain main themes run through both academic and activist statements:[14]

- Profits from illness must be abolished
- General policy and resource allocation must be managed at a national level, whereas detailed planning and administration must take place at regional and local levels, controlled by workers and other consumers
- A national health system, financed by progressive taxation, must provide comprehensive health services free to all citizens
- Relationships among health professionals and between them and their patients must be made less hierarchical and elitist and more egalitarian, by means of the redistribution of resources, altered policies of admission to training, and better communication

This is a distinctly socialist program, predicated upon major, though not necessarily violent social change. Radical medical thinkers see themselves as one focal point of a broad political movement that calls upon the nation to turn away from a society built on production and consumption to one organized around services, human survival, and self-realization.[15] The radical program is mainly on paper, but a half-step toward trying it out is being taken in the extraordinarily widespread and spontaneous free clinic movement.

The first modern free clinic was started by Dr. David Smith in 1967 in the Haight-Ashbury district of San Francisco to meet the desperate health needs of alienated and displaced youth.[16] Since then, hundreds of such clinics—30 in Los Angeles County alone—have been opened. Mostly urban, the clinics differ from each other because each is specifically designed to meet the needs of the population it serves. Supported unevenly by volunteer work, limited private and public funds, and patient donations, the clinics have been surprisingly durable. They stress egalitarianism, an open and consciously anti-bureaucratic style, patient participation, self-help, and free service.

The style of the clinics makes them acceptable to young people and members of minority groups who are apprehensive about bringing to established clinics or physicians' offices such problems as drug use, out-of-wedlock pregnancies, birth control, and venereal disease. As a recent analysis points out, in addition to meeting a distinct community need, the clinics "are also political acts and organizational reforms meant to influence education, care, and treatment."[17] Fragile creations, these clinics may change or disappear, but they have opened a crack in a remarkably rigid structure through which new light can enter.

Free clinics strive to bring health care workers and recipients together in an open encounter in which ordinary people are understood to have the right and the capacity to make decisions about their own health, with trained people present to help them rather than to administer to persons considered exclusively as "patients." In that important respect, the clinics may be forerunners of better patterns of human interaction in health care.

FRATERNAL WORK PATTERNS

Closer to the traditional mainstream of health practice, there are other changes that reassert basic needs for effective association and show that these needs can be met realistically in the context of urban health care in the United States. Group practice, family medicine, team care, consumer participation, and neighborhood health centers are some promising developments, and they have been discussed in earlier chapters. But these organizational forms are frequently advocated for pragmatic reasons that have little to do with human relationships and that, especially when they lead to unregulated growth, may actually increase the degree of depersonalization of our lives.

The shifting but continuous current in American life formed by the democratic idea of fraternity has been described by McWilliams.[18] He traces political thought that connects seventeenth-century white Puritanism with twentieth-century Black Pantherism and shows it to be an essential counterbalance to the excesses of liberty and equality. His redefinition of fraternity as a relation of affection founded on shared values and goals can be used as a touchstone to test the extent to which new forms of health care actually incorporate the fraternal principle.

Group practice

The motive that brings physicians together into group practices at first appears to be a straightforward economic one: they can share space, supporting services, and facilities; organize their work more efficiently; and compete more successfully for patients than they could as solo practitioners. The economic advantages of group practice for both physician and patient have been studied recently, with interest in them heightened by rapid increases in the cost of health care. The evidence is clear that prepaid group practice can effect savings along with broader coverage and acceptable quality and that there are probably similar but less pronounced advantages to fee-for-service group practice.[19] The more difficult question of whether group practice actually results in better health for participating patients is still unsettled, but the indications are that it may.[20]

The externally economic character of group practice is related to, but does not fully express other motives and forces also at work in a group. Among these are several that are explicitly fraternal. Mutual professional support and education is a prominent characteristic of group practice.[21, 22] Physicians who are attracted to this mode of practice give up some independence of action and agree to allow their professional behavior to be closely scrutinized by their peers in order to gain the reinforcement that comes from sharing knowledge and skill and from a closer identification with their colleagues.

Loyalty to the group is another common feature.[23] The loyalty of a new member is often established and tested during a trial period, which culminates either in a mutual agreement to separate or in a formal induction into membership, with specified rights and responsibilities.

The strength of the bond among physicians in a well-knit group not only enables them to work more freely with each other, with more trust, but can also provide them with a base from which to conduct more effective transactions at the professional borders of the group, with consultant physicians and with non-physician health workers.[24]

The importance of fraternal relationships in group practice is implicit in certain other characteristics, which are given less prominence because they do not contribute to or may even limit the economic advantages. Size is one such feature. Most groups in the United States are small, three-quarters consisting of three to five members, while 83 percent are simply organized as partnerships without the elaborate contractural agreements larger groups adopt.[25]

Another such characteristic is the internal strain that inevitably develops among physicians and others who work closely together. The successful working out of conflicts may greatly increase the morale of the group. In a group that has weathered the stresses of initial organization and adaptation, members are likely to feel that they have gone through an important personal experience, one that has made them into "a new breed."[26]

Does group practice also foster fraternal values by encouraging the physician to take a more personal interest in his patients and their families? Claims are made on both sides. Reviewing the question of how subscribers to large prepaid groups feel about the doctors and the services, Donabedian points out that dissatisfaction with the solo fee-for-service system is a frequent motive for enrollment in a group and that the great majority of active members express general satisfaction. In summary, however, he states "acceptability of prepaid group practice to broad segments of potential recipients and providers of care remains in considerable doubt."[27] Whether the patients of the more numerous small groups experience a more or less personal relationship with their physicians than they would with solo practitioners is even less clear. Nevertheless, small, manageable groups do provide a mechanism and a potential for change in the direction of better human relationships if consumers and providers wish to use them in this way, as well as for better coverage, better working relationships among physicians, and control of costs.

Team work

A leading problem of urban life is that advancing industrial technology, marked by accelerating automation and the tendency of industry to form ever larger complexes, has led to an increasing alienation of workers from the process as well as the product of their work (Chapter 3).

Research and experimentation on this problem have established some basic principles for the redesign of jobs. One of these is the need for better peer relationships among workers. "Most people are more satisfied to work as members of a group than in isolation. Workers prefer jobs that permit interaction and are more likely to quit jobs that prevent congenial peer relationships."[28] The kind of relationship needed to restore meaning to work is not simply friendly but includes understanding the jobs of co-workers, sharing in authority and decision-making within the group, and the opportunity to learn from and elicit the support of others. A second major feature of the new-style industrial production team is increased autonomy of the work group. This includes significant participation in decisions about methods, tasks, recruitment, leadership, scope of work, hours, incentive pay, and other vital matters long the prerogative of middle and upper echelons of management.

The widespread introduction of such policies throughout American industry is certain to be resisted in the name of efficiency by strong managers who perceive the social and economic consequences of decentralized decision-making, whereas the alert segments of organized labor, and consumers who are increasingly dissatisfied with the shoddy products of uninterested workers, will press for their adoption. The point here is that this lively dispute in industry shows that fraternal work patterns are proving to have an economic value and a measurable effect on the quality of the product.

If this is true for industrial production, how much more so for services, where attitudes of the worker impinge directly on the consumer! Neighborhood health centers, which were described in the previous chapter as experiments in social reform, may ultimately make their most important contribution as workshops in which to develop the team approach to primary health care.[29] Partly for reasons of social policy and partly out of economic necessity, the neighborhood health centers have become active producers and employers of new types of health worker, from the health advocate or outreach worker recruited from the population to be served, to persons trained at intermediate skill levels, designated as nurse practitioners, physicians' assistants, health associates, and others, the variety of which suggests how much real innovation is going on in the field.[30] New types of nonphysician health workers are being trained and employed in many other settings as well, usually in response to what is seen as a "health manpower" problem. The introduction of new categories of workers into a professional field already noted for its fragmentation must be justified. The neighborhood health center, by bringing old and new types of health workers together in a structured team with specific goals, should make it possible to determine whether such teams have personal and social as well as economic advantages.

At present, neighborhood center health care teams are too new to have produced the kind of evaluative data available for group practice. Accounts of the structure and function of teams in several centers, however, show that the idea of fraternal work relationships is prominent in their design.

Team members are expected to share common goals, and their combined effectiveness depends upon developing an explicit statement of objectives. As in group practice, peer relationships are critical, and team members, despite wide differences in social and educational background, are asked to allow their work to be reviewed and evaluated by other members, gaining, in the process, information, a sense of group solidarity, and a practical understanding of each other as persons and as professionals.[29, 31, 32]

Primary health care teams naturally encounter serious organizational problems. One that seems almost universal is defined, according to one's point of view, as the problem of leadership, or of the dominance of the physician. Non-physician team members, though acknowledging the more extensive training of the physician in diagnostic and medical therapeutic knowledge and skill, do not concede that he also automatically outranks other members in such skills as social perception, understanding of the family or the community, or judgment of human behavior. Working through these conflicts takes time and requires change in attitude and behavior on the part of physicians who are accustomed to the efficiency of a strongly hierarchical work relationship and on the part of nurses and others who have been trained as subordinates.[31, 32, 33] The interaction within health teams brings out another deep-seated problem, namely the stereotyped association of sex differences with specific health care roles. If female physicians and male nurses are to achieve full acceptance, the health care team is a good place to eliminate some of the barriers that now keep apart persons who should be able to work constructively together.

Small, close-knit professional teams are beginning to provide health services in many settings other than neighborhood health centers. The physician's traditional nurse-receptionist-secretary is being succeeded by an organized team in some solo and many small group practices. Emergency and ambulance services are being staffed by physicians' assistants specifically trained for the job who are skilled in working with nurses and physicians. Highly specialized hospital services, such as intensive coronary care, renal dialysis, and pulmonary disease units, function best when they are staffed by teams the members of which distribute the work according to training and skill and devote some time to improving their interaction.

Psychiatric and mental health services are adopting the therapeutic team, both in inpatient psychiatric units and in community mental health centers. One study of a clinical team in a psychiatric ward shows that such a work pattern enables team members to confront and begin to deal with the problems of task, process, social structure, and culture that can impede progress toward the common objective.[34] The authors of this study point out that the clinical psychiatric team is only one example of a general work pattern: "The small work group is a basic component of modern organizational life. Crucial tasks at every level of the organization are entrusted to work groups of various kinds: executive committees, staff meetings and committees with responsibility for policy review, budget planning, training, integration of services, and the like." Furthermore, they observe, "by and large, work groups do not work well . . . [and] the resultant costs to both the organization and the individual members are enormous. Despite the widespread dissatisfaction with work groups, relatively little effort has been given to the systematic analysis and improvement of their functioning."

Family medicine

The impressive growth of family practice since 1969 has been strongly motivated by the need, felt both by new health workers and by patients, for better human relationships than those commonly found in crowded public clinics or in the offices of many harried solo practitioners. Formal definitions of the role of the new family physician stress the transactional quality of what he does. He provides "first contact with the patient" and "personal medical care" and "assumes responsibility for the patient's total health care."[35] Building, as it must, on existing patterns of general practice, the new specialty has continued to tolerate solo practice. New residency programs, however, and some new textbooks increasingly stress the need for health care teams, usually with the family practitioner clearly designated as captain.[36, 37]

An important experiment in the provision of family medical care by interdisciplinary teams was conducted by Silver and others in the decade of the 1950's.[38, 39] The teams, consisting of an internist, a nurse, and a social worker, undertook to provide comprehensive care to 150 families belonging to a prepaid group.

Changes in these families were compared with those in a set of matched controls. This study was carefully planned and analyzed, and its findings are pertinent to the present development of family medicine. A major conclusion was that the "dignity and simplicity of good patient care can be enhanced by its appropriate organization" and that team practice can provide more intensive family care and more personal attention to the patient. Everything, of course, did not go according to plan. Efforts to redistribute tasks and to achieve balanced professional team work by the three members had to be modified when the patients expressed different expectations by turning to the doctor first and only secondarily to the nurse for care. Adaptations, however, could be made during the process of care by means of regular team conferences. In addition, the feasibility of regular conferences between health professionals and patients was demonstrated, and these discussions were judged to be more effective means of health maintenance than repetitive screening by annual physical examinations.

This study brings out the fact that family medicine ideally links one set of small group systems, namely, well-integrated professional teams, with another set, the diverse groups that comprise the modern family. The professional team must be small enough that patients can get to know its members. The relationship between team and family must work both ways, so that the health care system, in the form of identifiable persons, can become both responsive and accountable.

The teams in the Silver study also observed two important things about the mental health of the families they worked with. First, they found that there was a high degree of emotional distress in presumably normal families. Second, they recognized that many families had internal resources, which enabled them to cope with types of emotional problems that, in a minority of families, lead to disintegration or to heavy reliance on professional help. These findings reaffirmed that the family, as a social unit, can function in "fraternal" ways to support and care for ailing members. Skill in identifying and sustaining these strengths within the family can be one of the most effective tools available to the modern family practitioner (Chapter 4).

The diagnosis and treatment of the individual patient have been, for many years, the focal points of medical education and practice. Insofar as family and community relationships have been acknowledged, they have been seen as concentric environments surrounding the central transaction between doctor and patient.[40] A different conceptual model will be needed if family medicine is to mobilize and reinforce the latent creative, supportive, and therapeutic forces of the family. The change in perspective is radical and implies a basic change in medical education.[41] The social and behavioral sciences must be brought into a functional relationship with medicine in a manner analogous to the introduction of chemistry and microbiology a hundred years ago. Efforts to accomplish this are already demonstrating the fact that only a limited part of what psychology and sociology have learned about the family is applicable to medical practice, whereas much of what the effective family physician of the future will need to know remains to be discovered.[42] New techniques, ranging from family-based medical records to group therapy, will be needed to put the health care team into an informed, working relationship with groups of people living together as families. The need for new approaches is emphasized by a recent redefinition of the family as "any significant group of intimates with a history and a future."[41] Family medicine, therefore, provides another site for the development of collaborative work groups, organized with the specific objective of understanding and strengthening the healthy functioning of other persons in the context of their own living and working groups.

A question of size

A natural limit to the size of effective work and living groups is set by the capacity and need of individual human beings to form intimate relationships with others. This capacity varies, but most individuals find that when they are expected to relate closely to more than eight or ten people they begin to experience discomfort and to withdraw, partially or even, if the stress is great, completely. The extraneous forces of modern life, arising from such sources as accelerated transportation and communication and from economic pressure for the formation of larger, more "efficient" organizations, tend to expand relational groups beyond the size people find tolerable. Group medical practices, starting as a small cadre of friends or relatives, have had difficulty stopping their growth short of an institution the size of Mayo Clinic. A solo family practitioner, or two or three partners with a reliable office staff are often reluctant to form larger groups in spite of obvious advantages, because they fear the loss of familiar, intimate work relationships. We have learned to limit the size of a telephone number to the number of digits an average person can recall. We may also be able to determine what constitutes the limits of the social space within which most people can live and work with confidence and to use this dimension of space as a primary criterion in forming service groups, work teams, committees, hospital and nursing home units, and even home and group living arrangements.

The scale of human enterprise is a critical problem of our time that can be seen in nearly all institutions. Schumacher has put the issue vividly in his book, *Small Is Beautiful: A Study of Economics as if People Mattered.*[43] Basing his views on a radical critique of the assumptions implicit in modern economic theory, he points out how dangerous it is to omit from our calculations such essentials as the finiteness of natural resources and the need of human beings for work in a meaningful social context. "People," he says, "can be themselves only in small comprehensible groups. Therefore we must learn to think in terms of an articulated structure that can cope with a multiplicity of small-scale units. If economic thinking cannot grasp this it is useless." Small groups, he concedes, are not the solution to all contemporary problems, but since "today, we suffer from an almost universal idolatry of giantism, it is . . . necessary to insist on the virtues of smallness—where this applies." We must also reassert mastery over our tools. "We require from the scientists and technologists methods and equipment which are: cheap enough so that they are accessible to virtually everyone; suitable for small-scale application; and compatible with man's need for creativity."[44] At a time when the merits of national health insurance and prepaid group practice are being debated almost exclusively in "economic" (i.e., dollar cost) terms, Schumacher's larger conception of the social economy brings out of the shadows other costs that must be reckoned.

THE VALUE OF FRATERNITY

The small work and living group is an essential mediator between the individual and the institutions of mass society, but because of our historical preoccupation with the freedom of the individual we have underestimated its importance. The ambitious American has been ready to break away from his family, from his schoolmates, and his home town folks and to avoid strong personal connections, which might tie him down. The small group seems confining and provincial–a kind of heavy baggage that will only slow him down on the way to a new job and success.

From the perspective of equality, as well as from that of liberty, small groups can appear insignificant or even undemocratic. Inefficiency is the usual excuse for allowing an originally small group to be absorbed into a larger enterprise. Purely financial economies of scale are easier to effect in a larger hospital, a larger prepaid group practice, or in any other business. Worse, certain small groups can foster elitism, exclusiveness, and a monopoly of power. A small group "implies a necessary tension with loyalty to society at large."[45]

The disadvantages of the small fraternal group, therefore, can be magnified as we look at its juncture with individualism on the one hand and with egalitarianism on the other. Are there also advantages?

A strong case can be made for the proposition that the individual cannot fully realize his own potential except in close interaction with others. Animal experiments show that monkeys raised in isolation or with dummy "mothers" are stunted in their capacity to relate to other animals, to breed, and to rear offspring of their own.[46] Fraternity, according to McWilliams' extended definition, "is closely related to the development of 'ego identity,' since it includes a recognition of shortcomings and failure in the attainment of ultimate values, but provides the emotional encouragement and sense of worth ('assurance of identity') which makes it possible to endure such tensions without betraying one's own values."[45]

Clearly, the nuclear family group provides not only food and protection, but also the social and psychological support necessary to the early growth and development of the individual. Work and play groups in later life also foster continued education, communication of cognitive and behavioral skills, and novel sensory and intellectual stimuli in a non-threatening context that favors receptivity and response. Everyone recognizes the warm satisfaction that comes from a sense of belonging. The confidence with which we can turn to family or to colleagues and friends, renewed in family rituals, club meetings, and in the work conferences of healthy groups, is for most of us an essential nutrient for the sustained functioning of a mature personality. The small group can be a bridge to the larger social world of personal sustenance and a curb on egotistic drives. It can also serve to increase the amount of order in a disordered social system.

Perhaps the most vital function of fraternal work and living groups, however, will prove to be that of facilitating the behavior modification necessary for survival in the modern world without frustrating immutable biological and psychological needs of mankind. We know how urgent it is for us to learn to use less energy, to get along with fewer environmentally dangerous new products, and to protect the individual against the impact of the gigantic institutions a mass society needs in order to function. But we have great difficulty when it comes to acting on this knowledge, in large part because we lack the behavioral skills required to change established habits.

It is striking, for example, that the measures we have so far been able to devise for the prevention of the leading chronic diseases of our day are mainly forms of behavior modification. One type of prevention consists of controlling that behavior on which an individual may depend, such as smoking and drinking. Another has to do with establishing physical habits of regular, vigorous exercise and healthy relaxation. The most successful methods of inducing these changes have proved to be those that make use of the support and motivation of peers. Alcoholics Anonymous, group psychotherapy, sports clubs, and hundreds of other small group systems are being formed in increasing number. Whether such groups are organized specifically for health reasons or primarily as social and recreational units, they serve to reinforce the physical and psychological strengths of individual members by the means of a gratifying interaction with other persons with whom members share a fraternal bond, either of common social background and interests or the fellowship of illness.

A still more crucial function of the small group in the future of our society can be to create human-sized organizations in which average citizens once again participate in social and political action, with the direct reinforcement of visible results and the powerful motivation of comradeship. On the broadest social scale, such grass-roots organizations are urgently needed to counterbalance the steady trend toward centralized and autocratic power. The Sierra Club is a good example, since it both brings people together for political action to protect the environment and gives them the opportunity to associate with like-minded companions in such natural and biologically restorative activities as hiking and camping.

Many other examples could be cited. Common Cause and Ralph Nader's organization come immediately to mind as national plans to mobilize thousands of small local groups for concerted political action. The progress achieved in civil rights for minorities in the 1960's was initiated and led by church and lay groups, which used the appeal of brotherhood as a force for social action. In the field of health, consumer representation in neighborhood health centers and consumer-controlled prepaid group practices have already set examples that are beginning to have a wider effect in the writing of laws and the formation of new groups.

There is a danger, however, particularly evident in the "health maintenance organization" development, that the original conception of a truly fraternal group can be lost as growth occurs and as managerial ideology begins to prevail over humanitarian values. The kind of profit it is most reasonable to expect from a health service is not money but better health. Administrative decisions about size and the relationships between providers and recipients of service are likely to stifle rather than to nourish creative human relationships if they are based solely on considerations of cost.

It will not be easy to convince busy health workers, financially hard-pressed managers, and frustrated patients that they must invest extra time and effort in order to become active members of small work groups and to win significant autonomy for them. Decentralization of decision-making in a health care system of independent physicians and hierarchical hospitals will call for firmness, imagination, and persistence. Technological contributions to health care "accessible to everyone, suitable for small-scale application, and compatible with man's need for creativity" will not be provided without strong social demands for them, and the dangerous consequences of environmental exploitation will not come under control until enough people recognize them and are willing to participate with others in demanding restraints.

Faced with these tasks, we need new sources of strength. Mutually supportive groups of health workers, serving families whose strengths and autonomy they understand and reinforce, can be the model in the field of health care for new and healthier patterns of work and living. Fraternal values, after all, express the same human trait of gregariousness that inclines us to crowd together in cities. For all its attendant ills, urbanization offers the opportunity for collective action. Having built our cities carelessly, wastefully, and fraught with danger, we now have the chance to rebuild them as enduring human habitations, as a sustaining physical, biological, and social environment.

APPENDIX A

A central question in this study is whether the American city, as a whole, or in its parts, is a healthy or an unhealthy place to live. In order to arrive at an answer, we must begin by defining the terms. In searching for useful meanings of "city" and "health" it is immediately clear that these apparently simple terms in fact refer to complex phenomena with variable connotations arising from their intimate relationship to everyday human life. The most useful definitions will be those that are sufficiently operational to permit comparative measurements, but we must bear in mind that practical definitions may fail to express important social, personal, and esthetic qualities.

THE DEFINITION OF A CITY

In thinking about what cities are, the first impressions that come to mind may relate to their social characteristics–crowds, pace of life, dangers, opportunities. Sociologists, social historians, and a few psychologists have tried to formulate appropriate definitions. Wirth's verison, "a relatively large, dense, and permanent settlement of socially heterogeneous individuals," has been of use to sociology since 1938,[1] but a recent critique finds it inadequate and comes to the bleak conclusion that "a sociological definition of the city cannot be formulated."[2]

Toynbee, looking at the historical development of cities, offers a one-dimensional picture, "a settlement whose inhabitants cannot produce, within the city limits, all the food that they need."[3] Mumford, on the other hand, cautions that no single definition will apply to the city in all its manifestations,[4] and refers in various contexts to its functions as "magnet," "container," and "transformer." Psychologists have begun to formulate such dimensions as social "overloads" and the "atmosphere" of individual cities.[5] Though these social and psychological ideas undoubtedly touch on qualities that are related to health, they are not yet specific enough to serve as measures.

The most obvious fact about a city is that it is a geographic concentration of population. Opinions vary widely on how large a cluster of people must be before the area they occupy qualifies as a city. Prior to 1950, the United States census applied the term "urban" to places of 2,500 inhabitants or more. At this level, a simple distinction is being made between farm or rural on the one hand and all recognizable population clusters on the other. The process of urbanization, however, has produced highly complex settlements, which cannot be adequately described by a scale based on size alone. In assembling data for cities around the world, Davis selects as an index of urbanization the proportion of the population living in cities of 100,000 or more and comments that a unit of this size shows close correlation with other definitions.[6] Blumenfeld uses an operational definition that has an instinctive appeal for the modern commuter: "an area in which the travelling time from outskirts to center is no more than about 40 minutes." Such a city, in the United States today, contains about 500,000 people.[7]

A city is a "problem of organized complexity."[8] The definitions given so far have dealt with elements of population, land-use, and transportation. City planners, however, must also take into account the fact that, in developed countries in general and in the United States in particular, cities have been formed by commercial, economic, and industrial forces[9]—"a transaction-maximizing system."[10] The train, the automobile, and the truck have allowed the central city, which was originally compact, to expand centrifugally. Smaller "ekistic" units have dispersed first, and cities have come to be ringed by suburban residential areas. The character of these areas is changing as larger units, such as shopping centers and light manufacturing, follow the population away from downtown in order to maximize the transactions of production and consumption. An economist notes that "elite services," including hospitals, tend to remain in the central city, in contrast with retail and wholesale trade and manufacturing, which are dispersing more rapidly. This pattern is more pronounced in the older cities of the United States.[11]

Another characteristic must be recognized in the search for a definition that can be related to health. The political structure of a city, in spite of, or even because of its often arbitrary boundaries and lack of relationship to modern population and economic structure, has a great influence on the distribution and availability of health services. Historically, the United States has produced some "cities" that contain only a fraction of the population of a metropolitan region, whereas a few cities, such as Los Angeles and San Diego, include large tracts of thinly populated land. This inconsistency suggests that a better working unit might be the county. Counties are also significant political units, and they tend to be a little more uniform in size throughout the country.

It is an interesting commentary on the economic and industrial nature of American cities that the most widely accepted definition in recent years is that established by the Bureau of the Budget. The Standard Metropolitan Statistical Area (SMSA) is a county or a group of contiguous counties containing at least one city of 50,000 inhabitants or more. Contiguous counties are included in an SMSA if, according to specified criteria, they are essentially metropolitan in character and are socially and economically integrated with the central city.[12] This definition comprehends population size, political structure, and social and economic relationships. It has the advantage that the counties containing the central cities represent the most highly urbanized places, whereas the remainder of the SMSA counties can be taken as a mainly suburban population. These non-central city SMSA counties will be referred to as suburban counties, though they are about one-third urban and two-thirds rural in terms of the earlier definitions. The appropriateness of the term is demonstrated by the fact that these counties are not only adjacent to cities and functionally related to them but are also intermediate in population density, with the highest proportion of high-income residents and the lowest proportion of low-income residents.[13] Metropolitan counties, containing urban plus suburban counties, can be contrasted with non-metropolitan counties outside the SMSA. For certain kinds of data, the non-metropolitan counties can also be subdivided into farm and non-farm populations on the basis of occupation and residence. Table 6.1 shows the relative sizes of these population units.

Precise identification of the suburban population is complicated by the fact that two different categories have been used in reporting the census, one based on counties and the other consisting of different population-size groups. More than two-thirds of the U.S. population in 1970 (68.6 percent) lived in the Standard Metropolitan Statistical Areas. Within these SMSA's, counties that contained a central city accounted for 53.3 percent of the total U.S. population. Most of the persons living in these central city counties (31.4 percent of the U.S. population) lived in the central city itself and were classified as "urban." The remaining 21.9 percent of the U.S. population that lived in these central city counties may be considered residents of the inner suburban ring. Also identifiable as suburban are the 15.3 percent of the U.S. population who lived in contiguous SMSA counties that did not contain a central city. Thus, 31.4 percent of the U.S. population may be considered to be urban (i.e., living in cities of 50,000 or more), 37.2 percent suburban, and the remaining 31.4 percent who lived outside SMSA counties non-metropolitan.

Because national mortality data by residence are tabulated by county, it is evident from the above that mortality figures for central city counties are diluted by some suburban data, and that the only available measure of suburban mortality consists of data from SMSA counties that have no central city. In Appendix B and in the textual figures, therefore, metropolitan counties without central cities are used to represent the suburban population.

HEALTH INDICATORS

Having arrived at a definition we can use to relate health characteristics to the degree of urbanization, we must next examine the types of information about health that are available and assess the quality of the data. Unfortunately, we do not have complete and accurate information about health, and better health statistics are an urgent national need.[14]

Three main kinds of information have been collected in a sufficiently uniform way to be used as a basis for general statements about urban health in the United States. These are mortality rates, based on death certificates and census, and rates of morbidity and use of services, obtained from national health examination and health interview surveys. These are the fundamental data used throughout the book, supplemented by information from other surveys, special studies, and many other sources.

Almost every death in the United States is recorded on a standard death certificate. Since these records are collected by governmental units, which differ in some ways from the units used for collecting census information, the calculation of mortality rates is complicated. For this and other reasons the complete publication of annual vital statistics has lagged by three or four years, and the annual reports do not relate deaths to area of residence in any detail. Mortality rates, subdivided according to the SMSA definition of metropolitan areas, have been published for the 1950 census[15] and have been calculated but only partially published for the 1960 census.[16] A study of differential mortality in the United States, which deals with differences related to residence in 1960, has recently been published by Kitagawa and Hauser.[17] The mortality rates presented in Fig. 1.1 and subsequent figures are based on tabulations of the number of deaths in the United States by 30 causes of death, by county of residence, by race, and by sex, for the three years 1969 through 1971.[18] The population used for calculating rates is that provided by the 1970 census. Detailed tables are presented in Appendix B.

Mortality rates are marred by errors of completeness and accuracy, as discussed by Grove and Hetzel.[19] Death registration in the United States is probably over 95 percent complete. The most significant deficiencies for the present study are those that differ from one area to another. Death certificate diagnoses may differ considerably from autopsy diagnoses (6 to 29 percent), and there is some evidence that the quality of diagnosis, as judged by this standard, is less satisfactory among rural practitioners.[20] Infant mortality rates present special problems, since the registration of live births is less complete in rural than in urban areas, so that low weight infants who die immediately after birth are probably underreported or reported as fetal deaths.[21, 22]

A death is assigned to the "usual place of residence." The people of the United States have often been described as restless and mobile. How mobile they are is a critical question for determining relationships between health and place of residence. The length of exposure to city air and the duration of access to urban health services may bear an important relationship to how these and other factors influence health. Fortunately, the question of population mobility has been thoroughly studied by Taeuber and coworkers.[23] Special questions about residence were added to the Current Population Survey of a national sample comprising 35,000 households in May, 1958. Two-thirds of the adult population were found to have lived in the "current place" for 10 years or more and 95 percent for 1 year or more. Shorter residence times were most prevalent among the young adult population, and residential stability increased with age. At ages 75 and over, 82 percent had not moved for 10 years or more.

This is a very different image of the mobility of the American population from the one called up by the well-known census finding that 20 percent of persons change residence every year.[24] The difference is explained by the fact that in Taeuber's study "place" is defined as anywhere within the limits of an urban place, city, town, village or borough, or, for rural residents, within a county. Thus we can assume with considerable confidence that most people have been exposed to the environment of the city, suburb, town, or rural area in which they live for several years at least. Since most deaths and much morbidity occurs among older people, who are also the most stable residentially, relationships between residence and mortality become even more significant.

The age distribution of the United States population differs by residential areas. Non-metropolitan counties, for example, had 11.3 percent aged 65 and over in 1970, whereas this age group included only 8.0 percent of the residents of metropolitan non-central city (suburban) counties (Table 6.1). For this reason, the standard epidemiological technique of direct age-adjustment is used in presenting mortality data, taking the 1940 United States population as a base in order to permit comparison with data for previous decades.

Information about morbidity and use of services has been collected on systematic samples of the civilian, non-institutional population of the United States since 1957. Health interviews provide a continuous series of estimates,[25] and health examinations, using mobile units, give periodic information on a national basis.[26, 27] The design of these surveys and such source limitations as sampling, lack of cooperation, errors of memory, and population mobility are analyzed in individual publications of the National Center for Health Statistics.[28] In general, errors that can be identified and estimated do not show any striking relationship to residence. As the process of data collection continues, and as methods are refined, the reappearance of similar patterns in repeated surveys increases confidence in their significance. Sampling errors can be estimated most precisely, and the estimates reported in this study are those that are "significant" in that they show differences greater than those that can be explained by chance errors in sampling (5 percent level).

APPENDIX B

ables of Average Annual Deaths and Crude and Age-Adjusted Death Rates for Selected Causes of Death (U.S.), 1959-1961 (Tables 29 and 30) and 1969-71 ables 1 through 28), by County of Residence, Sex, and Color. (Rates per 0,000 Population; Age-Adjustment to 1940 U.S. Population.)

ble o.	Cause of Death	ICDA No. (8th Rev.)	Figure
	All causes		1.1
	Tuberculosis, all forms	010-019	1.2
	Other infective and parasitic diseases	Remainder of 000-136	6.1
	Malignant neoplasms, including neoplasms of lymphatic and hematopoietic tissue	140-209	1.4
	Malignant neoplasm of digestive organs and peritoneum	150-159	1.5
	Malignant neoplasm of respiratory system	160-163	1.3
	Malignant neoplasm of breast	174	1.5
	Malignant neoplasm of genital organs	180-187	1.6
	Malignant neoplasm of urinary organs	188, 189	1.5
	Leukemia	204-207	1.6
	Diabetes mellitus	250	6.9
	Diseases of heart	390-398, 402, 404, 410-429	1.7
	Active rheumatic fever and chronic rheumatic heart disease	390-398	1.7
	Hypertensive heart disease with or without renal disease	402, 404	6.7
	Ischemic heart disease	410-413	1.7
	Hypertension	400, 401, 403	6.7
	Cerebrovascular disease	430-438	6.8
	Influenza and pneumonia	470-474, 480-486	1.2
	Bronchitis, emphysema, and asthma	490-493	6.10
	Peptic ulcer	531-533	6.3
	Cirrhosis of liver	571	3.2
	Nephritis and nephrosis	580-584	6.7
	Congenital anomalies	740-759	6.5
	Certain causes of mortality in early infancy	760-769.2, 769.4-772, 774-778	3.1
	Motor vehicle accidents	E810-E823	6.4
	All other accidents	E800-E807, E825-E949	3.1
	Suicide	E950-E959	3.3
	Homicide	E960-E978	3.3
	Appendicitis (1959-61)	(7th Rev.) 550-553	6.2
	Malignant neoplasm of cervix uteri (1959-61)	(7th Rev.) 171	6.6

asterisk (*) by an age-adjusted rate in the tables means that more than one-half of age-specific rates upon which that figure is based had fewer than 20 deaths in the age up.

erage numbers of annual deaths were obtained by averaging over a 3-year period; totals ome categories differ slightly from the sums of subcategories, due to rounding.

Table 1
All causes

	TOTAL	Male	Female	WHITE Total	WHITE Male	WHITE Female	ALL OTHER Total	ALL OTHER Male	ALL OTHER Female
United States									
Deaths	1,923,521	1,078,912	844,609	1,685,163	943,385	741,778	238,358	135,527	102,831
Crude rate	946.5	1,090.6	809.7	946.2	1,085.5	813.4	948.2	1,127.5	783.9
Age-adjusted rate	710.8	931.2	527.7	674.7	891.4	495.7	996.5	1,251.0	780.0
Metropolitan Counties with Central Cities									
Deaths	1,023,839	566,743	457,097	872,511	480,438	392,072	151,329	86,304	65,024
Crude rate	944.4	1,083.0	815.0	951.3	1,081.7	828.8	906.5	1,090.3	740.8
Age-adjusted rate	724.6	953.0	541.4	679.9	902.7	503.4	997.6	1,261.0	777.3
Metropolitan Counties without Central Cities									
Deaths	237,723	132,028	105,695	222,360	123,257	99,101	15,362	8,769	6,594
Crude rate	753.8	853.3	657.9	749.7	846.7	656.3	817.6	959.9	683.0
Age-adjusted rate	659.6	856.0	498.0	645.4	841.0	485.3	904.6	1,123.7	713.6
Non-Metropolitan Counties									
Deaths	661,959	380,142	281,817	590,292	339,687	250,605	71,667	40,454	31,213
Crude rate	1,046.1	1,221.5	876.3	1,040.8	1,216.2	870.6	1,091.7	1,268.0	925.1
Age-adjusted rate	713.8	934.9	519.7	682.6	902.5	489.8	1,023.2	1,267.7	808.8

Table 2
Tuberculosis, all forms, 010-019 (ICDA, 8th Rev.)

					WHITE			*ALL OTHER*	
	TOTAL	*Male*	*Female*	*Total*	*Male*	*Female*	*Total*	*Male*	*Female*
United States									
Deaths	5,095	3,638	1,457	3,562	2,569	993	1,533	1,069	464
Crude rate	2.5	3.7	1.4	2.0	3.0	1.1	6.1	8.9	3.5
Age-adjusted rate	2.1	3.3	1.1	1.6	2.5	0.8	7.0	10.7	3.9
Metropolitan Counties with Central Cities									
Deaths	3,132	2,259	873	2,046	1,493	553	1,085	766	320
Crude rate	2.9	4.3	1.6	2.2	3.4	1.2	6.5	9.7	3.6
Age-adjusted rate	2.5	4.0	1.3	1.8	2.9	0.9	7.7	11.9	4.1
Metropolitan Counties without Central Cities									
Deaths	467	327	140	376	262	114	91	65	26
Crude rate	1.5	2.1	0.9	1.3	1.8	0.8	4.8	7.2	2.7
Age-adjusted rate	1.4	2.2	0.8	1.2	1.8*	0.6*	5.7*	8.9*	2.9*
Non-Metropolitan Counties									
Deaths	1,496	1,052	444	1,140	814	326	356	238	119
Crude rate	2.4	3.4	1.4	2.0	2.9	1.1	5.4	7.4	3.5
Age-adjusted rate	1.8	2.7	1.0	1.4	2.2	0.8	5.8	8.3	3.8

Table 3
Other infective and parasitic diseases, Remainder of 000-136 (ICDA, 8th Rev.)

				WHITE			*ALL OTHER*		
	TOTAL	*Male*	*Female*	*Total*	*Male*	*Female*	*Total*	*Male*	*Female*
United States									
Deaths	10,934	5,687	5,247	8,396	4,336	4,060	2,538	1,351	1,187
Crude rate	5.4	5.7	5.0	4.7	5.0	4.5	10.1	11.2	9.0
Age-adjusted rate	4.6	5.1	4.1	3.9	4.4	3.5	9.5	10.6	8.5
Metropolitan Counties with Central Cities									
Deaths	5,809	3,041	2,768	4,377	2,285	2,092	1,432	756	676
Crude rate	5.4	5.8	4.9	4.8	5.1	4.4	8.6	9.6	7.7
Age-adjusted rate	4.6	5.3	4.1	3.9	4.5	3.4	8.5	9.6	7.6
Metropolitan Counties without Central Cities									
Deaths	1,243	628	615	1,087	549	538	156	79	77
Crude rate	3.9	4.1	3.8	3.7	3.8	3.6	8.3	8.7	8.0
Age-adjusted rate	3.6	4.0	3.4	3.3	3.7	3.1	7.9*	8.3*	7.5*
Non-Metropolitan Counties									
Deaths	3,882	2,018	1,864	2,932	1,503	1,429	950	516	434
Crude rate	6.1	6.5	5.8	5.2	5.4	5.0	14.5	16.2	12.9
Age-adjusted rate	5.0	5.5	4.7	4.1	4.5	3.8	12.5	13.9	11.3

Table 4

Malignant neoplasms, including neoplasms of lymphatic and hematopoietic tissues, 140-209 (ICDA, 8th Rev.)

				WHITE			ALL OTHER		
	TOTAL	Male	Female	Total	Male	Female	Total	Male	Female
United States									
Deaths	330,407	180,059	150,348	296,016	160,517	135,499	34,390	19,542	14,849
Crude rate	162.6	182.0	144.1	166.2	184.7	148.6	136.8	162.6	113.2
Age-adjusted rate	129.0	156.8	107.9	126.6	153.6	106.2	151.1	187.4	121.1
Metropolitan Counties with Central Cities									
Deaths	182,063	98,380	83,683	158,956	85,155	73,801	23,107	13,225	9,882
Crude rate	167.9	188.0	149.2	173.3	191.7	156.0	138.4	167.1	112.6
Age-adjusted rate	135.0	166.3	112.2	131.4	161.3	110.0	160.5	203.2	125.8
Metropolitan Counties without Central Cities									
Deaths	43,962	23,524	20,438	41,595	22,196	19,399	2,367	1,328	1,039
Crude rate	139.4	152.0	127.2	140.2	152.5	128.5	126.0	145.3	107.7
Age-adjusted rate	129.0	155.4	109.6	128.0	154.1	108.9	148.8	181.3	121.6
Non-Metropolitan Counties									
Deaths	104,382	58,155	46,227	95,466	53,166	42,300	8,916	4,989	3,928
Crude rate	165.0	186.9	143.7	168.3	190.3	146.9	135.8	156.4	116.4
Age-adjusted rate	120.1	144.1	100.3	119.0	143.1	99.2	132.1	156.6	111.3

Table 5
Malignant neoplasm of digestive organs and peritoneum, 150-159 (ICDA, 8th Rev.)

				WHITE			*ALL OTHER*		
	TOTAL	*Male*	*Female*	*Total*	*Male*	*Female*	*Total*	*Male*	*Female*
United States									
Deaths	94,534	50,552	43,982	84,376	44,610	39,766	10,159	5,942	4,217
Crude rate	46.5	51.1	42.2	47.4	51.3	43.6	40.4	49.4	32.1
Age-adjusted rate	34.9	43.2	28.3	33.9	41.6	27.7	44.2	57.1	33.3
Metropolitan Counties with Central Cities									
Deaths	52,717	28,303	24,413	45,784	24,223	21,561	6,933	4,080	2,852
Crude rate	48.6	54.1	43.5	49.9	54.5	45.6	41.5	51.5	32.5
Age-adjusted rate	37.1	47.1	29.5	35.6	44.9	28.6	48.2	63.1	35.9
Metropolitan Counties without Central Cities									
Deaths	12,325	6,507	5,818	11,645	6,107	5,538	680	400	280
Crude rate	39.1	42.1	36.2	39.3	41.9	36.7	36.2	43.8	29.0
Age-adjusted rate	35.1	42.9	29.0	34.7	42.3	28.8	42.7	54.9	32.3
Non-Metropolitan Counties									
Deaths	29,493	15,742	13,751	26,947	14,280	12,666	2,546	1,462	1,085
Crude rate	46.6	50.6	42.8	47.5	51.1	44.0	38.8	45.8	32.1
Age-adjusted rate	31.5	37.7	26.2	31.0	37.0	26.0	36.2	45.8	28.0

Table 6
Malignant neoplasm of respiratory system, 160-163 (ICDA, 8th Rev.)

					WHITE			*ALL OTHER*	
	TOTAL	*Male*	*Female*	*Total*	*Male*	*Female*	*Total*	*Male*	*Female*
United States									
Deaths	69,484	56,196	13,288	62,418	50,408	12,010	7,066	5,788	1,278
Crude rate	34.2	56.8	12.7	35.0	58.0	13.2	28.1	48.2	9.7
Age-adjusted rate	28.3	50.3	10.2	27.8	49.5	10.1	31.9	57.0	10.7
Metropolitan Counties with Central Cities									
Deaths	39,043	31,182	7,861	34,044	27,089	6,956	4,999	4,093	905
Crude rate	36.0	59.6	14.0	37.1	61.0	14.7	29.9	51.7	10.3
Age-adjusted rate	30.0	53.9	11.2	29.2	52.4	11.1	35.3	63.5	11.8
Metropolitan Counties without Central Cities									
Deaths	9,299	7,415	1,884	8,801	7,006	1,795	498	409	89
Crude rate	29.5	47.9	11.7	29.7	48.1	11.9	26.5	44.8	9.2
Age-adjusted rate	28.2	49.6	10.6	28.0	49.2	10.6	32.1	57.0	10.7*
Non-Metropolitan Counties									
Deaths	21,142	17,599	3,543	19,572	16,313	3,259	1,570	1,286	284
Crude rate	33.4	56.5	11.0	34.5	58.4	11.3	23.9	40.3	8.4
Age-adjusted rate	25.7	45.7	8.2	25.8	45.9	8.2	24.5	43.4	8.2

Table 7
Malignant neoplasm of breast, 174 (ICDA, 8th Rev.)

					WHITE			*ALL OTHER*	
	TOTAL	*Male*	*Female*	*Total*	*Male*	*Female*	*Total*	*Male*	*Female*
United States									
Deaths	29,759	275	29,484	27,216	245	26,972	2,543	31	2,512
Crude rate	14.6	0.3	28.3	15.3	0.3	29.6	10.1	0.3	19.1
Age-adjusted rate	12.5	0.3	22.9	12.5	0.3*	23.0	11.7	0.3*	21.3
Metropolitan Counties with Central Cities									
Deaths	16,897	147	16,750	15,163	128	15,035	1,734	20	1,715
Crude rate	15.6	0.3	29.9	16.5	0.3	31.8	10.4	0.2	19.5
Age-adjusted rate	13.3	0.3*	24.1	13.4	0.3*	24.3	12.3	0.3*	22.3
Metropolitan Counties without Central Cities									
Deaths	4,348	39	4,309	4,160	37	4,123	188	2	186
Crude rate	13.8	0.2	26.8	14.0	0.3	27.3	10.0	0.2	19.3
Age-adjusted rate	13.2	0.3*	24.4	13.2	0.3*	24.4	12.1	0.2*	22.4
Non-Metropolitan Counties									
Deaths	8,514	89	8,425	7,893	80	7,813	621	9	611
Crude rate	13.5	0.3	26.2	13.9	0.3	27.1	9.5	0.3	18.1
Age-adjusted rate	10.8	0.2*	20.1	10.8	0.2*	20.2	10.2	0.3*	18.7

Table 8

Malignant neoplasm of genital organs, 180-187 (ICDA, 8th Rev.)

					WHITE			*ALL OTHER*	
	TOTAL	*Male*	*Female*	*Total*	*Male*	*Female*	*Total*	*Male*	*Female*
United States									
Deaths	41,405	18,336	23,069	35,628	15,667	19,961	5,777	2,669	3,108
Crude rate	20.4	18.5	22.1	20.0	18.0	21.9	23.0	22.2	23.7
Age-adjusted rate	15.6	14.4	17.6	14.7	13.5	16.7	25.0	24.3	26.0
Metropolitan Counties with Central Cities									
Deaths	21,896	9,322	12,573	18,325	7,715	10,609	3,571	1,607	1,964
Crude rate	20.2	17.8	22.4	20.0	17.4	22.4	21.4	20.3	22.4
Age-adjusted rate	15.8	14.5	17.9	14.7	13.3	16.8	24.7	24.7*	25.4
Metropolitan Counties without Central Cities									
Deaths	5,128	2,161	2,967	4,752	1,996	2,756	376	165	211
Crude rate	16.3	14.0	18.5	16.0	13.7	18.3	20.0	18.1	21.9
Age-adjusted rate	14.7	14.0	16.6	14.3	13.6	16.1	23.4	22.0*	25.2
Non-Metropolitan Counties									
Deaths	14,381	6,853	7,528	12,551	5,955	6,596	1,830	897	932
Crude rate	22.7	22.0	23.4	22.1	21.3	22.9	27.9	28.1	27.6
Age-adjusted rate	15.9	14.5	17.9	14.9	13.7	16.8	26.3	24.3*	28.4

Table 9

Malignant neoplasm of urinary organs, 188, 189 (ICDA, 8th Rev.)

				WHITE			ALL OTHER		
	TOTAL	*Male*	*Female*	*Total*	*Male*	*Female*	*Total*	*Male*	*Female*
United States									
Deaths	15,233	10,175	5,058	14,010	9,412	4,598	1,223	763	460
Crude rate	7.5	10.3	4.8	7.9	10.8	5.0	4.9	6.3	3.5
Age-adjusted rate	5.6	8.6	3.3	5.6	8.7	3.2	5.3	7.3	3.7
Metropolitan Counties with Central Cities									
Deaths	8,275	5,497	2,778	7,468	4,998	2,470	807	498	308
Crude rate	7.6	10.5	5.0	8.1	11.3	5.2	4.8	6.3	3.5
Age-adjusted rate	5.8	9.0	3.3	5.8	9.2	3.3	5.6	7.7	3.9
Metropolitan Counties without Central Cities									
Deaths	2,057	1,395	662	1,974	1,341	633	83	54	29
Crude rate	6.5	9.0	4.1	6.7	9.2	4.2	4.4	5.9	3.0
Age-adjusted rate	5.8	9.2	3.2	5.9	9.3	3.3	5.1*	7.4*	3.3*
Non-Metropolitan Counties									
Deaths	4,901	3,283	1,618	4,568	3,073	1,495	333	211	122
Crude rate	7.7	10.6	5.0	8.1	11.0	5.2	5.1	6.6	3.6
Age-adjusted rate	5.3	7.8	3.1	5.3	8.0	3.1	4.7*	6.4*	3.2*

Table 10
Leukemia, 204-207 (8th Rev.)

					WHITE			*ALL OTHER*	
	TOTAL	*Male*	*Female*	*Total*	*Male*	*Female*	*Total*	*Male*	*Female*
United States									
Deaths	14,470	8,197	6,274	13,346	7,556	5,791	1,124	641	483
Crude rate	7.1	8.3	6.0	7.5	8.7	6.4	4.5	5.3	3.7
Age-adjusted rate	5.8	7.3	4.6	5.9	7.4	4.7	4.7	5.8	3.8
Metropolitan Counties with Central Cities									
Deaths	7,463	4,139	3,324	6,739	3,723	3,017	723	416	307
Crude rate	6.9	7.9	5.9	7.3	8.4	6.4	4.3	5.3	3.5
Age-adjusted rate	5.7	7.1	4.6	5.8	7.3	4.7	4.7	6.0	3.7
Metropolitan Counties without Central Cities									
Deaths	1,975	1,123	852	1,898	1,080	818	78	43	34
Crude rate	6.3	7.3	5.3	6.4	7.4	5.4	4.1	4.7	3.6
Age-adjusted rate	5.8	7.3	4.6	5.8	7.4	4.6	4.5*	5.3*	3.8*
Non-Metropolitan Counties									
Deaths	5,032	2,935	2,098	4,709	2,753	1,956	323	181	142
Crude rate	8.0	9.4	6.5	8.3	9.9	6.8	4.9	5.7	4.2
Age-adjusted rate	5.9	7.4	4.6	6.0	7.6	4.7	4.7	5.6	3.9

Table 11
Diabetes Mellitus, 250 (ICDA, 8th Rev.)

	TOTAL	*Male*	*Female*	*WHITE* *Total*	*WHITE* *Male*	*WHITE* *Female*	*ALL OTHER* *Total*	*ALL OTHER* *Male*	*ALL OTHER* *Female*
United States									
Deaths	38,374	15,675	22,698	32,444	13,553	18,891	5,930	2,122	3,808
Crude rate	18.9	15.8	21.8	18.2	15.6	20.7	23.6	17.7	29.0
Age-adjusted rate	14.0	13.5	14.4	12.7	12.7	12.7	25.9	20.6	30.4
Metropolitan Counties with Central Cities									
Deaths	20,334	8,272	12,062	16,587	6,901	9,685	3,747	1,371	2,376
Crude rate	18.8	15.8	21.5	18.1	15.5	20.5	22.4	17.3	27.1
Age-adjusted rate	14.2	13.9	14.4	12.6	12.9	12.4	26.1	21.3	30.0
Metropolitan Counties without Central Cities									
Deaths	4,766	1,949	2,817	4,387	1,816	2,570	379	133	247
Crude rate	15.1	12.6	17.5	14.8	12.5	17.0	20.2	14.5	25.5
Age-adjusted rate	13.3	12.8	13.5	12.7	12.6	12.7	23.8	18.2*	28.5
Non-Metropolitan Counties									
Deaths	13,274	5,454	7,820	11,470	4,835	6,635	1,803	619	1,185
Crude rate	21.0	17.5	24.3	20.2	17.3	23.0	27.5	19.4	35.1
Age-adjusted rate	14.1	13.2	14.8	13.0	12.6	13.2	26.7	20.3	32.1

Table 12

Diseases of heart, 390-398, 402, 404, 410-429 (ICDA, 8th Rev.)

				WHITE			*ALL OTHER*		
	TOTAL	*Male*	*Female*	*Total*	*Male*	*Female*	*Total*	*Male*	*Female*
United States									
Deaths	739,392	419,826	319,565	669,804	382,112	287,692	69,588	37,714	31,874
Crude rate	363.8	424.4	306.4	376.1	439.7	315.5	276.8	313.8	243.0
Age-adjusted rate	253.1	349.8	173.7	248.2	348.4	166.0	292.3	356.5	238.5
Metropolitan Counties with Central Cities									
Deaths	391,716	218,468	173,247	348,027	194,892	153,135	43,688	23,576	20,112
Crude rate	361.3	417.5	308.9	379.4	438.8	323.7	261.7	297.8	229.1
Age-adjusted rate	257.5	357.0	178.7	251.2	355.0	169.3	296.4	361.4	242.4
Metropolitan Counties without Central Cities									
Deaths	93,526	52,982	40,545	88,894	50,447	38,447	4,632	2,535	2,098
Crude rate	296.6	342.4	252.4	299.7	346.5	254.6	246.5	277.5	217.3
Age-adjusted rate	249.6	342.3	173.0	247.8	342.4	169.9	280.8	342.6	227.9
Non-Metropolitan Counties									
Deaths	254,150	148,376	105,773	232,882	136,773	96,110	21,267	11,604	9,664
Crude rate	401.6	476.8	328.9	410.6	489.7	333.9	324.0	363.7	286.4
Age-adjusted rate	248.5	343.4	166.5	244.6	342.8	159.7	288.6	350.4	235.8

Table 13

Active rheumatic fever and chronic rheumatic heart disease, 390-398 (ICDA, 8th Rev.)

				WHITE			ALL OTHER		
	TOTAL	Male	Female	Total	Male	Female	Total	Male	Female
United States									
Deaths	14,988	6,897	8,091	13,637	6,256	7,381	1,352	642	710
Crude rate	7.4	7.0	7.8	7.7	7.2	8.1	5.4	5.3	5.4
Age-adjusted rate	6.4	6.5	6.2	6.3	6.5	6.2	6.2	6.4	6.0
Metropolitan Counties with Central Cities									
Deaths	8,715	3,903	4,812	7,771	3,455	4,316	945	449	496
Crude rate	8.0	7.5	8.6	8.5	7.8	9.1	5.7	5.7	5.7
Age-adjusted rate	6.9	7.0	6.8	6.9	7.0	6.8	6.6	6.9	6.4
Metropolitan Counties without Central Cities									
Deaths	2,124	957	1,167	2,029	915	1,114	95	42	53
Crude rate	6.7	6.2	7.3	6.8	6.3	7.4	5.1	4.6	5.5
Age-adjusted rate	6.5	6.4	6.6	6.6	6.5	6.6	6.1*	5.7*	6.4*
Non-Metropolitan Counties									
Deaths	4,149	2,037	2,112	3,837	1,886	1,951	312	151	161
Crude rate	6.6	6.5	6.6	6.8	6.8	6.8	4.8	4.7	4.8
Age-adjusted rate	5.4	5.7	5.1	5.4	5.7	5.1	5.2	5.4	5.2

Table 14

Hypertensive heart disease with or without renal disease, 402, 404 (ICDA, 8th Rev.)

				WHITE			ALL OTHER		
	TOTAL	*Male*	*Female*	*Total*	*Male*	*Female*	*Total*	*Male*	*Female*
United States									
Deaths	15,109	6,533	8,576	12,082	5,108	6,974	3,027	1,425	1,602
Crude rate	7.4	6.6	8.2	6.8	5.9	7.6	12.0	11.9	12.2
Age-adjusted rate	5.0	5.3	4.7	4.1	4.4	3.9	13.0	13.7	12.4
Metropolitan Counties with Central Cities									
Deaths	7,542	3,259	4,283	5,659	2,368	3,291	1,883	891	992
Crude rate	7.0	6.2	7.6	6.2	5.3	7.0	11.3	11.3	11.3
Age-adjusted rate	4.9	5.3	4.6	3.9	4.2	3.6	13.0	13.8	12.2
Metropolitan Counties without Central Cities									
Deaths	1,625	687	938	1,420	599	821	205	88	117
Crude rate	5.2	4.4	5.8	4.8	4.1	5.4	10.9	9.6	12.2
Age-adjusted rate	4.2	4.4	3.9	3.7	4.0	3.5*	12.7	12.0*	13.3*
Non-Metropolitan Counties									
Deaths	5,941	2,587	3,355	5,002	2,141	2,862	939	446	493
Crude rate	9.4	8.3	10.4	8.8	7.7	9.9	14.3	14.0	14.6
Age-adjusted rate	5.3	5.5	5.1	4.6	4.8	4.4	12.9	13.5	12.3

Table 15
Ischemic heart disease, 410-413 (ICDA, 8th Rev.)

	TOTAL	Male	Female	WHITE Total	WHITE Male	WHITE Female	ALL OTHER Total	ALL OTHER Male	ALL OTHER Female
United States									
Deaths	670,262	384,756	285,506	611,954	352,962	258,992	58,308	31,794	26,514
Crude rate	329.8	388.9	273.7	343.6	406.1	284.0	232.0	264.5	202.1
Age-adjusted rate	227.6	319.5	152.2	225.3	321.0	146.9	243.7	299.9	196.6
Metropolitan Counties with Central Cities									
Deaths	357,118	201,274	155,844	320,208	181,194	139,014	36,910	20,079	16,831
Crude rate	329.4	384.6	277.9	349.1	407.9	293.9	221.1	253.7	191.7
Age-adjusted rate	232.7	327.7	157.4	229.4	329.1	150.8	250.1	308.1	201.9
Metropolitan Counties without Central Cities									
Deaths	85,553	49,031	36,522	81,668	46,887	34,781	3,885	2,144	1,740
Crude rate	271.3	316.9	227.3	275.4	322.1	230.3	206.7	234.7	180.3
Age-adjusted rate	227.3	316.6	153.5	226.8	318.1	151.6	234.6	289.8	187.2
Non-Metropolitan Counties									
Deaths	227,591	134,451	93,140	210,078	124,881	85,197	17,513	9,570	7,943
Crude rate	359.7	432.0	289.6	370.4	447.1	296.0	266.8	300.0	235.4
Age-adjusted rate	220.9	310.1	144.0	219.5	312.2	139.4	234.6	286.3	190.4

Table 16
Hypertension, 400, 401, 403 (ICDA, 8th Rev.)

				WHITE			ALL OTHER		
	TOTAL	*Male*	*Female*	*Total*	*Male*	*Female*	*Total*	*Male*	*Female*
United States									
Deaths	8,179	4,205	3,974	6,243	3,194	3,049	1,935	1,011	924
Crude rate	4.0	4.3	3.8	3.5	3.7	3.3	7.7	8.4	7.0
Age-adjusted rate	2.9	3.5	2.4	2.2	2.8	1.8	8.7	10.1	7.6
Metropolitan Counties with Central Cities									
Deaths	4,054	2,050	2,004	2,912	1,466	1,447	1,142	585	557
Crude rate	3.7	3.9	3.6	3.2	3.3	3.1	6.8	7.4	6.3
Age-adjusted rate	2.8	3.4	2.4	2.1	2.6	1.7	8.0	9.1	7.1
Metropolitan Counties without Central Cities									
Deaths	916	463	453	797	400	397	118	63	56
Crude rate	2.9	3.0	2.8	2.7	2.7	2.6	6.3	6.9	5.8
Age-adjusted rate	2.4	3.0	2.1	2.2	2.7*	1.8*	7.5*	8.6*	6.6*
Non-Metropolitan Counties									
Deaths	3,209	1,692	1,517	2,534	1,328	1,205	675	364	311
Crude rate	5.1	5.4	4.7	4.5	4.8	4.2	10.3	11.4	9.2
Age-adjusted rate	3.2	3.9	2.7	2.5	3.1	2.1	10.7	12.6	9.1

Table 17
Cerebrovascular disease, 430-438 (ICDA, 8th Rev.)

	TOTAL	*Male*	*Female*	*WHITE* *Total*	*Male*	*Female*	*ALL OTHER* *Total*	*Male*	*Female*
United States									
Deaths	207,812	93,974	113,838	181,806	81,617	100,189	26,007	12,357	13,650
Crude rate	102.3	95.0	109.1	102.1	93.9	109.9	103.5	102.8	104.1
Age-adjusted rate	66.0	73.8	60.0	61.4	69.3	55.4	108.2	115.5	102.0
Metropolitan Counties with Central Cities									
Deaths	104,070	45,588	58,482	89,496	38,770	50,725	14,574	6,817	7,757
Crude rate	96.0	87.1	104.3	97.6	87.3	107.2	87.3	86.1	88.4
Age-adjusted rate	64.2	71.2	59.0	59.4	66.5	54.1	98.7	104.4	93.9
Metropolitan Counties without Central Cities									
Deaths	23,975	10,610	13,365	22,343	9,835	12,508	1,632	774	858
Crude rate	76.0	68.6	83.2	75.3	67.6	82.8	86.9	84.8	88.8
Age-adjusted rate	60.5	67.2	55.4	58.6	65.3	53.4	97.9	103.3	93.4
Non-Metropolitan Counties									
Deaths	79,767	37,777	41,991	69,967	33,011	36,956	9,800	4,756	5,035
Crude rate	126.1	121.4	130.6	123.4	118.2	128.4	149.3	149.4	149.2
Age-adjusted rate	70.8	79.6	63.4	65.4	74.2	58.2	129.8	140.7	120.4

Table 18

Influenza and pneumonia, 470-474, 480-486 (ICDA, 8th Rev.)

				WHITE			*ALL OTHER*		
	TOTAL	*Male*	*Female*	*Total*	*Male*	*Female*	*Total*	*Male*	*Female*
United States									
Deaths	62,766	34,867	27,899	53,045	29,055	23,990	9,721	5,812	3,909
Crude rate	30.9	35.2	26.7	29.8	33.4	26.3	38.7	48.4	29.8
Age-adjusted rate	21.9	28.5	16.6	19.7	25.8	15.0	37.6	49.7	27.4
Metropolitan Counties with Central Cities									
Deaths	33,989	18,940	15,049	27,790	15,172	12,618	6,199	3,768	2,432
Crude rate	31.4	36.2	26.8	30.3	34.2	26.7	37.1	47.6	27.7
Age-adjusted rate	22.9	30.5	17.1	20.3	27.1	15.3	38.2	51.7	27.0
Metropolitan Counties without Central Cities									
Deaths	7,134	3,853	3,282	6,565	3,523	3,042	569	329	240
Crude rate	22.6	24.9	20.4	22.1	24.2	20.1	30.3	36.1	24.9
Age-adjusted rate	18.5	24.0	14.4	17.8	23.1	13.8	30.7	39.2	23.5
Non-Metropolitan Counties									
Deaths	21,642	12,074	9,568	18,690	10,359	8,331	2,953	1,715	1,237
Crude rate	34.2	38.8	29.8	33.0	37.1	28.9	45.0	53.8	36.7
Age-adjusted rate	21.7	27.5	16.9	19.7	25.2	15.2	38.4	48.2	29.9

Table 19
Bronchitis, emphysema, and asthma, 490-493 (ICDA, 8th Rev.)

				WHITE			ALL OTHER		
	TOTAL	Male	Female	Total	Male	Female	Total	Male	Female
United States									
Deaths	30,772	24,106	6,666	28,666	22,598	6,068	2,106	1,508	598
Crude rate	15.1	24.4	6.4	16.1	26.0	6.7	8.4	12.5	4.6
Age-adjusted rate	11.5	20.3	4.7	11.6	20.8	4.6	9.1	14.3	4.9
Metropolitan Counties with Central Cities									
Deaths	15,931	12,163	3,768	14,500	11,156	3,344	1,431	1,006	424
Crude rate	14.7	23.2	6.7	15.8	25.1	7.1	8.6	12.7	4.8
Age-adjusted rate	11.3	20.0	5.0	11.4	20.4	4.9	9.8	15.2	5.3
Metropolitan Counties without Central Cities									
Deaths	3,637	2,856	781	3,503	2,752	751	134	104	30
Crude rate	11.5	18.5	4.9	11.8	18.9	5.0	7.1	11.3	3.1
Age-adjusted rate	10.5	18.9	4.1	10.6	19.2	4.1	8.4*	14.1*	3.6*
Non-Metropolitan Counties									
Deaths	11,204	9,088	2,117	10,663	8,690	1,973	541	398	143
Crude rate	17.7	29.2	6.6	18.8	31.1	6.9	8.2	12.5	4.2
Age-adjusted rate	12.2	21.4	4.5	12.5	22.2	4.5	8.1	12.5	4.3

Table 20
Peptic ulcer, 531-533 (ICDA, 8th Rev.)

					WHITE			*ALL OTHER*	
	TOTAL	*Male*	*Female*	*Total*	*Male*	*Female*	*Total*	*Male*	*Female*
United States									
Deaths	8,680	5,750	2,930	7,867	5,190	2,677	813	560	253
Crude rate	4.3	5.8	2.8	4.4	6.0	2.9	3.2	4.7	1.9
Age-adjusted rate	3.3	5.0	1.9	3.2	4.9	1.9	3.6	5.5	2.0
Metropolitan Counties with Central Cities									
Deaths	4,761	3,127	1,633	4,222	2,759	1,463	538	368	170
Crude rate	4.4	6.0	2.9	4.6	6.2	3.1	3.2	4.6	1.9
Age-adjusted rate	3.4	5.3	2.0	3.3	5.2	1.9	3.7	5.7	2.1
Metropolitan Counties without Central Cities									
Deaths	1,025	663	362	975	627	348	50	36	14
Crude rate	3.3	4.3	2.3	3.3	4.3	2.3	2.7	3.9	1.5
Age-adjusted rate	2.9	4.4	1.8	2.9	4.3	1.8	3.2*	4.9*	1.7*
Non-Metropolitan Counties									
Deaths	2,894	1,960	934	2,669	1,803	866	225	156	68
Crude rate	4.6	6.3	2.9	4.7	6.5	3.0	3.4	4.9	2.0
Age-adjusted rate	3.2	4.9	1.8	3.2	4.9	1.8	3.5	5.3*	1.9*

Table 21
Cirrhosis of liver, 571 (ICDA, 8th Rev.)

					WHITE			*ALL OTHER*	
	TOTAL	*Male*	*Female*	*Total*	*Male*	*Female*	*Total*	*Male*	*Female*
United States									
Deaths	31,024	20,147	10,877	26,168	17,193	8,976	4,856	2,955	1,901
Crude rate	15.3	20.4	10.4	14.7	19.8	9.8	19.3	24.6	14.5
Age-adjusted rate	14.5	20.0	9.7	13.3	18.6	8.6	23.7	31.2	17.3
Metropolitan Counties with Central Cities									
Deaths	20,787	13,544	7,243	16,873	11,132	5,741	3,914	2,412	1,502
Crude rate	19.2	25.9	12.9	18.4	25.1	12.1	23.4	30.5	17.1
Age-adjusted rate	18.3	25.6	12.1	16.6	23.6	10.6	28.2	37.9	20.0
Metropolitan Counties without Central Cities									
Deaths	3,649	2,300	1,348	3,363	2,122	1,241	286	178	107
Crude rate	11.6	14.9	8.4	11.3	14.6	8.2	15.2	19.5	11.1
Age-adjusted rate	11.5	15.4	8.2	11.1	14.9	7.8	18.7	24.9*	13.3*
Non-Metropolitan Counties									
Deaths	6,589	4,303	2,286	5,932	3,939	1,993	656	364	292
Crude rate	10.4	13.8	7.1	10.5	14.1	6.9	10.0	11.4	8.7
Age-adjusted rate	9.5	13.0	6.4	9.2	12.8	5.9	13.0	15.1	11.1

Table 22
Nephritis and nephrosis, 580-584 (ICDA, 8th Rev.)

					WHITE			*ALL OTHER*	
	TOTAL	*Male*	*Female*	*Total*	*Male*	*Female*	*Total*	*Male*	*Female*
United States									
Deaths	8,912	4,808	4,105	6,630	3,616	3,014	2,283	1,192	1,091
Crude rate	4.4	4.9	3.9	3.7	4.2	3.3	9.1	9.9	8.3
Age-adjusted rate	3.6	4.3	3.0	2.8	3.5	2.3	10.1	11.6	8.9
Metropolitan Counties with Central Cities									
Deaths	4,671	2,487	2,184	3,217	1,731	1,486	1,454	756	698
Crude rate	4.3	4.8	3.9	3.5	3.9	3.1	8.7	9.5	8.0
Age-adjusted rate	3.6	4.4	3.0	2.7	3.4	2.2	10.1	11.6	8.8
Metropolitan Counties without Central Cities									
Deaths	943	513	430	809	444	365	133	69	65
Crude rate	3.0	3.3	2.7	2.7	3.1	2.4	7.1	7.5	6.7
Age-adjusted rate	2.8	3.4	2.3	2.5	3.1	2.0	8.3	9.2*	7.5*
Non-Metropolitan Counties									
Deaths	3,299	1,808	1,491	2,603	1,440	1,163	695	367	328
Crude rate	5.2	5.8	4.6	4.6	5.2	4.0	10.6	11.5	9.7
Age-adjusted rate	3.9	4.6	3.2	3.2	3.9	2.6	10.9	12.2	9.9

Table 23
Congenital anomalies, 740-759 (ICDA, 8th Rev.)

	TOTAL	Male	Female	WHITE Total	WHITE Male	WHITE Female	ALL OTHER Total	ALL OTHER Male	ALL OTHER Female
United States									
Deaths	16,596	8,863	7,734	14,101	7,529	6,572	2,495	1,333	1,162
Crude rate	8.2	9.0	7.4	7.9	8.7	7.2	9.9	11.1	8.9
Age-adjusted rate	7.5	8.0	7.1	7.5	7.9	7.0	7.8	8.5	7.2
Metropolitan Counties with Central Cities									
Deaths	8,951	4,753	4,199	7,270	3,858	3,412	1,682	895	787
Crude rate	8.3	9.1	7.5	7.9	8.7	7.2	10.1	11.3	9.0
Age-adjusted rate	7.6	8.0	7.1	7.5	7.9	7.1	7.9	8.6	7.3
Metropolitan Counties without Central Cities									
Deaths	2,340	1,248	1,092	2,163	1,157	1,006	177	91	86
Crude rate	7.4	8.1	6.8	7.3	7.9	6.7	9.4	10.0	8.9
Age-adjusted rate	6.9	7.3	6.5	6.8	7.2	6.4	7.6*	8.1*	7.2*
Non-Metropolitan Counties									
Deaths	5,305	2,862	2,443	4,669	2,515	2,154	636	347	289
Crude rate	8.4	9.2	7.6	8.2	9.0	7.5	9.7	10.9	8.9
Age-adjusted rate	7.8	8.4	7.3	7.8	8.4	7.3	7.7	8.5*	6.9*

Table 24

Certain causes of mortality in early infancy, 760-769.2, 769.4-772, 774-778 **(*ICDA*, *8th Rev.*)**

					WHITE			*ALL OTHER*	
	TOTAL	*Male*	*Female*	*Total*	*Male*	*Female*	*Total*	*Male*	*Female*
United States									
Deaths	41,623	24,394	17,229	31,033	18,376	12,657	10,590	6,018	4,572
Crude rate	20.5	24.7	16.5	17.4	21.1	13.9	42.1	50.1	34.9
Age-specific rate (under 1 year/1,000)	11.9	13.7	10.1	10.5	12.2	8.8	19.5	22.0	16.9
Metropolitan Counties with Central Cities									
Deaths	23,087	13,461	9,626	15,778	9,333	6,445	7,309	4,128	3,181
Crude rate	21.3	25.7	17.2	17.2	21.0	13.6	43.8	52.1	36.2
Age-specific rate (under 1 year/1,000)	12.3	14.0	10.4	10.4	12.0	8.7	20.3	22.8	17.8
Metropolitan Counties without Central Cities									
Deaths	5,348	3,168	2,181	4,592	2,731	1,861	757	437	320
Crude rate	17.0	20.5	13.6	15.5	18.8	12.3	40.3	47.8	33.1
Age-specific rate (under 1 year/1,000)	10.0	11.5	8.3	9.2	10.7	7.7	19.0	22.0	16.1
Non-Metropolitan Counties									
Deaths	13,188	7,766	5,423	10,664	6,312	4,351	2,525	1,453	1,071
Crude rate	20.8	25.0	16.9	18.8	22.6	15.1	38.5	45.6	31.8
Age-specific rate (under 1 year/1,000)	12.2	14.1	10.3	11.4	13.2	9.5	17.6	20.2	14.9

Table 25

Motor vehicle accidents, E810-E823 (ICDA, 8th Rev.)

				WHITE			ALL OTHER		
	TOTAL	Male	Female	Total	Male	Female	Total	Male	Female
United States									
Deaths	54,935	39,445	15,490	47,578	33,967	13,611	7,357	5,478	1,879
Crude rate	27.0	39.9	14.9	26.7	39.1	14.9	29.3	45.6	14.3
Age-adjusted rate	27.6	41.4	14.6	27.0	40.2	14.5	31.9	51.5	14.9
Metropolitan Counties with Central Cities									
Deaths	23,882	16,907	6,975	20,127	14,154	5,973	3,755	2,753	1,002
Crude rate	22.0	32.3	12.4	21.9	31.9	12.6	22.5	34.8	11.4
Age-adjusted rate	22.2	33.2	12.1	21.9	32.4	12.1	24.2	38.7	11.8
Metropolitan Counties without Central Cities									
Deaths	7,247	5,187	2,060	6,676	4,764	1,912	571	423	148
Crude rate	23.0	33.5	12.8	22.5	32.7	12.7	30.4	46.3	15.3
Age-adjusted rate	24.1	36.0	13.0	23.5	35.1	12.8	33.2	52.1	16.1
Non-Metropolitan Counties									
Deaths	23,807	17,351	6,455	20,775	15,049	5,726	3,031	2,302	729
Crude rate	37.6	55.8	20.1	36.6	53.9	19.9	46.2	72.2	21.6
Age-adjusted rate	38.9	58.5	19.9	37.5	56.0	19.5	53.7	86.7	23.6

Table 26
All other accidents, E800-E807, E825-E949

					WHITE			*ALL OTHER*	
	TOTAL	*Male*	*Female*	*Total*	*Male*	*Female*	*Total*	*Male*	*Female*
United States									
Deaths	59,886	40,108	19,778	49,826	32,941	16,885	10,059	7,167	2,893
Crude rate	29.5	40.5	19.0	28.0	37.9	18.5	40.0	59.6	22.1
Age-adjusted rate	26.2	39.3	13.9	24.0	36.0	12.8	41.5	64.7	21.1
Metropolitan Counties with Central Cities									
Deaths	30,285	19,725	10,560	24,401	15,557	8,844	5,884	4,168	1,716
Crude rate	27.9	37.7	18.8	26.6	35.0	18.7	35.2	52.7	19.5
Age-adjusted rate	24.8	36.7	14.0	22.6	33.1	12.9	37.1	57.7	19.4
Metropolitan Counties without Central Cities									
Deaths	6,963	4,640	2,322	6,300	4,143	2,157	663	497	166
Crude rate	22.1	30.0	14.5	21.2	28.5	14.3	35.3	54.4	17.2
Age-adjusted rate	20.8	30.7	11.6	19.8	29.0	11.3	36.8	58.9	16.6
Non-Metropolitan Counties									
Deaths	22,638	15,743	6,896	19,126	13,241	5,885	3,512	2,501	1,011
Crude rate	35.8	50.6	21.4	33.7	47.4	20.4	53.5	78.4	30.0
Age-adjusted rate	31.3	48.3	14.9	28.7	44.4	13.5	54.6	85.3	26.7

Table 27
Suicide, E950-E959 (ICDA, 8th Rev.)

	TOTAL	Male	Female	WHITE Total	WHITE Male	WHITE Female	ALL OTHER Total	ALL OTHER Male	ALL OTHER Female
United States									
Deaths	23,312	16,449	6,863	21,891	15,426	6,465	1,421	1,022	399
Crude rate	11.5	16.6	6.6	12.3	17.8	7.1	5.7	8.5	3.0
Age-adjusted rate	11.7	17.2	6.8	12.3	18.0	7.3	6.7	10.4	3.5
Metropolitan Counties with Central Cities									
Deaths	12,949	8,729	4,220	11,934	8,016	3,918	1,015	714	301
Crude rate	11.9	16.7	7.5	13.0	18.0	8.3	6.1	9.0	3.4
Age-adjusted rate	12.2	17.3	7.7	12.9	18.2	8.3	7.1	10.9	3.9
Metropolitan Counties without Central Cities									
Deaths	3,166	2,164	1,002	3,081	2,102	979	85	62	23
Crude rate	10.0	14.0	6.2	10.4	14.4	6.5	4.5	6.8	2.3
Age-adjusted rate	10.6	15.1	6.5	10.9	15.5	6.8	5.4*	8.3*	2.7*
Non-Metropolitan Counties									
Deaths	7,197	5,556	1,642	6,876	5,309	1,567	321	247	74
Crude rate	11.4	17.9	5.1	12.1	19.0	5.4	4.9	7.7	2.2
Age-adjusted rate	11.5	18.0	5.5	12.0	18.8	5.7	6.1	9.9	2.7*

Table 28
Homicide, E960-E978 (ICDA, 8th Rev.)

					WHITE			*ALL OTHER*	
	TOTAL	*Male*	*Female*	*Total*	*Male*	*Female*	*Total*	*Male*	*Female*
United States									
Deaths	17,037	13,419	3,619	7,793	5,845	1,948	9,244	7,574	1,670
Crude rate	8.4	13.6	3.5	4.4	6.7	2.1	36.8	63.0	12.7
Age-adjusted rate	9.4	15.3	3.8	4.8	7.4	2.3	43.4	76.8	14.5
Metropolitan Counties with Central Cities									
Deaths	11,754	9,355	2,399	4,782	3,617	1,164	6,972	5,737	1,235
Crude rate	10.8	17.9	4.3	5.2	8.1	2.5	41.8	72.5	14.1
Age-adjusted rate	11.9	19.7	4.6	5.6	8.8	2.6	47.5	85.4	15.4
Metropolitan Counties without Central Cities									
Deaths	1,343	1,021	322	870	632	238	473	390	84
Crude rate	4.3	6.6	2.0	2.9	4.3	1.6	25.2	42.7	8.7
Age-adjusted rate	4.7	7.4	2.2	3.2	4.8	1.7	29.0	50.3	9.7*
Non-Metropolitan Counties									
Deaths	3,940	3,043	897	2,142	1,596	546	1,798	1,447	352
Crude rate	6.2	9.8	2.8	3.8	5.7	1.9	27.4	45.3	10.4
Age-adjusted rate	7.2	11.5	3.2	4.3	6.5	2.1	36.8	62.8	13.6

Table 29
Appendicitis, 550-553 (ICDA, 7th Rev.)

	TOTAL	Male	Female	WHITE Total	WHITE Male	WHITE Female	ALL OTHER Total	ALL OTHER Male	ALL OTHER Female
United States									
Deaths	1,844	1,156	688	1,526	968	558	317	187	130
Crude rate	1.0	1.3	0.8	1.0	1.2	0.7	1.5	1.9	1.2
Age-adjusted rate	0.9	1.2	0.6	0.8	1.1	0.6	1.7	2.1	1.3
Metropolitan Counties with Central Cities									
Deaths	946	595	351	761	489	272	185	106	79
Crude rate	1.0	1.3	0.7	1.0	1.3	0.7	1.5	1.8	1.3
Age-adjusted rate	0.9	1.2	0.6	0.8	1.1	0.5	1.7	2.1*	1.4*
Metropolitan Counties without Central Cities									
Deaths	156	93	63	143	88	55	13	5	8
Crude rate	0.7	0.9	0.6	0.7	0.9	0.5	1.2	1.0	1.3
Age-adjusted rate	0.7	0.9	0.5*	0.7	0.9*	0.5*	1.3*	1.1*	1.4*
Non-Metropolitan Counties									
Deaths	741	467	274	622	391	231	119	76	43
Crude rate	1.1	1.4	0.8	1.1	1.3	0.8	1.6	2.1	1.2
Age-adjusted rate	0.9	1.2	0.7	0.9	1.1	0.6	1.7	2.3*	1.2*

Table 30
Malignant neoplasm of cervix uteri, 171 (ICDA, 7th Rev.)

	TOTAL			WHITE			ALL OTHER		
	TOTAL	Male	Female	Total	Male	Female	Total	Male	Female
United States									
Deaths	8,464	—	8,464	6,779	—	6,779	1,685	—	1,685
Crude rate	4.7	—	9.3	4.3	—	8.4	8.2	—	16.0
Age-adjusted rate	4.4	—	8.4	3.8	—	7.3	9.6	—	18.5
Metropolitan Counties with Central Cities									
Deaths	4,526	—	4,526	3,503	—	3,503	1,023	—	1,023
Crude rate	4.9	—	9.6	4.4	—	8.6	8.5	—	16.4
Age-adjusted rate	4.5	—	8.5	3.8	—	7.3	9.8	—	18.9
Metropolitan Counties without Central Cities									
Deaths	768	—	768	688	—	688	80	—	80
Crude rate	3.5	—	7.0	3.3	—	6.6	7.1	—	13.9
Age-adjusted rate	3.5	—	6.8	3.3	—	6.4	8.2*	—	16.0*
Non-Metropolitan Counties									
Deaths	3,170	—	3,170	2,588	—	2,588	582	—	582
Crude rate	4.8	—	9.6	4.4	—	8.8	8.0	—	15.7
Age-adjusted rate	4.5	—	8.8	4.0	—	7.8	9.5	—	18.4

REFERENCES AND NOTES

CHAPTER 1

1. Hippocrates, *The Theory and Practice of Medicine* (New York: Philosophical Library, 1964).
2. D. Hunter, *The Diseases of Occupations,* 4th ed. (Boston: Little, Brown, 1969), pp. 90-146.
3. R. A. Kehoe, Standards for the prevention of occupational lead poisoning. *Archives of Environmental Health* 23, 245-48 (1971).
4. V. F. Guinee, Lead poisoning. *American Journal of Medicine* 52, 283-88 (1972).
5. Hunter, *Diseases of Occupations,* p. 272.
6. L. A. Blanksma, H. K. Sachs, E. F. Murray, and M. J. O'Connell, Incidence of high blood lead levels in Chicago children. *Pediatrics* 44, 661-67 (1969).
7. U.S. Department of Health, Education and Welfare, Public Health Service, Division of Air Pollution, Working Group on Lead Contamination, *Survey of Lead in the Atmosphere of Three Urban Communities,* P.H.S. Publication No. 999-AP-12 (Washington, D.C.: U.S. Government Printing Office, 1965).
8. R. J. Caprio, H. L. Margulis, and M. M. Joselow, Lead absorption in children and its relationship to urban traffic densities. *Archives of Environmental Health* 28, 195-97 (1974).

9. J. S. Lin-Fu, Undue absorption of lead among children: A new look at an old problem. *New England Journal of Medicine* 286, 702-10 (1972).
10. C. J. Cohen, G. N. Bowers, and M. L. Lepow, Epidemiology of lead poisoning: A comparison between urban and rural children. *Journal of the American Medical Association* 226, 1430-33 (1973).
11. U.S. Department of Health, Education and Welfare, Public Health Service, Medical aspects of childhood lead poisoning. *Pediatrics* 48, 464-68 (1971).
12. J. F. Gilsinn, *Estimates of the Nature and Extent of Lead Paint Poisoning in the United States,* U.S. Department of Commerce, National Bureau of Standards, Tech Note 746 (Washington, D.C.: U.S. Government Printing Office, 1972).
13. J. J. Chisholm, Jr., Lead poisoning. *Scientific American* 224, 15-23 (1971).
14. A. A. Browder, M. M. Joselow, and D. B. Louria, The problem of lead poisoning. *Medicine* 52, 121-39 (1973).
15. M. E. Osband and J. R. Tobin, Lead paint exposure in migrant labor camps. *Pediatrics* 49, 604-6 (1972).
16. J. Storck, *Report of the Twentieth Anniversary Conference of the United States National Committee on Vital and Health Statistics,* U.S. Department of Health, Education and Welfare, National Center for Health Statistics, P.H.S. Publication 1000, Series 4, No. 13 (Rockville, Maryland, 1970).
17. T. Rodman and F. H. Sterling, *Pulmonary Emphysema and Related Lung Diseases* (St. Louis: C. V. Mosby, 1969), pp. 3-23.
18. R. S. Chapman, C. M. Shy, J. F. Finklea, D. E. House, H. E. Goldberg, and C. G. Hays, Chronic respiratory disease: in military inductees and parents of schoolchildren. *Archives of Environmental Health* 27, 138-42 (1973).
19. J. R. Goldsmith, Effects of air pollution on human health. *Air Pollution,* ed. A. C. Stern, vol. 1, 2nd ed. (New York: Academic Press, 1968), pp. 547-616.
20. U.S. Department of Health, Education and Welfare, Public Health Service, *Air Quality Criteria for Sulfur Oxides,* National Air Pollution Control Administration Publication No. AP-50 (Washington, D.C.: U.S. Government Printing Office, January, 1969), pp. 117-49.
21. S. M. Ayres and M. E. Buehler, The effects of urban air pollution on health. *Clinical Pharmacology and Therapeutics* 11, 337-71 (1970).
22. I. T. T. Higgins, Effects of sulfur oxides and particulates on health. *Archives of Environmental Health* 22, 584-90 (1971).
23. J. R. Goldsmith, The new airborne disease: Community air pollution. *California Medicine* 113, 13-20 (1970).
24. R. Doll, Atmospheric pollution. *Monographs on Neoplastic Disease at Various Sites,* ed. D. W. Smithers (Edinburgh: E & S Livingstone,

1958–), vol. 1, *Carcinoma of the Lung,* ed. J. R. Bignall (1958), pp. 81-94.

25. J. Clemmesen, Statistical studies in the aetiology of malignant neoplasms. *Pathologiotica et Microbiologia Scandanavia,* Suppl. 174, 319, 543 (1965).
26. Goldsmith, *Effects of Air Pollution on Human Health,* p. 568.
27. M. Lerner and O. W. Anderson, *Health Progress in the United States, 1900–1960* (Chicago: University of Chicago Press, 1963).
28. M. H. Griswold, C. S. Wilder, S. G. Cutler, and E. S. Pollack, *Cancer in Connecticut, 1935–1951,* Connecticut State Department of Health (Hartford, Conn., 1955), pp. 97-101.
29. W. Haenszel, S. C. Marcus, and E. G. Zimmerer, *Cancer Morbidity in Urban and Rural Iowa,* Public Health Monograph No. 37, P.H.S. Publication No. 462 (Washington, D.C.: U.S. Government Printing Office, 1956).
30. M. I. Levin, W. Haenzel, B. E. Carroll, P. R. Gerhardt, V. H. Handy, and S. C. Ingraham, II, Cancer incidence in urban and rural areas of New York state. *Journal of the National Cancer Institute* 24, 1243-57 (1960).
31. A. B. Ford, Urban Factors in Relation to Cancer (Paper presented to Epidemiology Section, American Public Health Association, New Orleans, Louisiana, October 22, 1974).
32. H. R. Menck, J. T. Casagrande, and B. E. Henderson, Industrial air pollution: Possible effect on lung cancer. *Science* 183, 210-11 (1974).
33. G. Dean, Lung cancer among white South Africans. *British Medical Journal* 2, 852-57 (1959).
34. E. C. Hammond and D. Horn, "Smoking and death rates—Report on forty-four months of follow-up of 187,783 men: Death rates by cause. *Journal of the American Medical Association* 166, 1294-1308 (1958).
35. E. C. Hammond, O. Auerbach, D. Kirman, and L. Garfinkel, Effect of cigarette smoking on dogs. I. Design of experiment, mortality, and findings in lung parenchyma. *Archives of Environmental Health* 21, 740-53 (December, 1970).
36. O. Auerbach, E. C. Hammond, D. Kirman, and L. Garfinkel, Effects of cigarette smoking on dogs. II. Pulmonary neoplasms. *Archives of Environmental Health* 21, 754-68 (December, 1970).
37. P. Stocks, On the relations between atmospheric pollution in urban and rural localities and mortality from cancer, bronchitis and pneumonia, with particular reference to 3:4 benzopyrene, beryllium, molybdenum, vanadium and arsenic. *British Journal of Cancer* 14, 397-418 (1960).
38. P. Buell, J. E. Dunn, Jr., and L. Breslow, Cancer of the lung and Los Angeles-type air pollution. *Cancer* 20, 2139-47 (1967).
39. E. L. Wynder, J. Kmet, N. Dungal, and M. Segi, An epidemiological investigation of gastric cancer. *Cancer* 16, 1461-96 (1963).
40. U.S. Department of Commerce, Bureau of the Census, *Historical Sta-*

tistics of the United States, Colonial Times to 1957, Series L 155-163, (Washington, D.C.: U.S. Government Printing Office, 1960).

41. M. O. Amdur, Toxicologic appraisal of particulate matter, oxides sulfur, and sulfuric acid. *Journal of the Air Pollution Control Association* 19, 638-44 (1969).
42. R. J. Hickey, D. E. Boyce, E. B. Harner, and R. C. Clelland, Ecological statistical studies concerning environmental pollution and chronic disease. *IEEE Transactions on Geoscience Electronics* GE-8, 186-202 (1970).
43. L. D. Zeidberg, R. J. M. Horton, and E. Landau, The Nashville air pollution study: V. Mortality from diseases of the respiratory system in relation to air pollution. *Archives of Environmental Health* 15, 214-224 (1967).
44. P. K. Mueller and M. Hitchcock, Air quality criteria toxicological appraisal for oxidants, nitrogen oxides, and hydrocarbons. *Journal of the Air Pollution Control Association* 19, 12-21 (1969).
45. H. F. Stokinger and D. L. Coffin, Biologic effects of air pollutants. *Air Pollution: vol. I. Air Pollution and Its Effects,* ed. A. C. Stern (New York: Academic Press, 1968), pp. 446-546.
46. W. Winkelstein, Jr., and S. Kantor, Stomach cancer: Positive association with suspended particulate air pollution. *Archives of Environmental Health* 18, 544-47 (1969).
47. W. Winkelstein, Jr., and S. Kantor, Respiratory symptoms and air pollution in an urban population of northeastern United States. *Archives of Environmental Health* 18, 760-67 (1969).
48. R. M. Hagstrom, H. A. Sprague, and E. Landau, The Nashville air pollution study: VII. Mortality from cancer in relation to air pollution. *Archives of Environmental Health* 15, 237-48 (1967).
49. J. Higginson, Present trends in cancer epidemiology. *Canadian Cancer Conference, Proceedings of the Eighth Canadian Cancer Conference,* ed. J. F. Morgan (New York: Pergamon Press, 1968), pp. 40-75.
50. W. C. Hueper, *Occupational and Environmental Cancers of the Respiratory System* (New York: Springer-Verlag, 1966).
51. I. J. Selikoff and E. C. Hammond, Environmental epidemiology; III. Community effects of nonoccupational environmental asbestos exposure. *American Journal of Public Health* 58, 1658-66 (1968).
52. E. Sawicki, Airborne carcinogens and allied compounds. *Archives of Environmental Health* 14, 46-53 (1967).
53. D. B. Clayson, *Chemical Carcinogenesis* (Boston: Little, Brown, 1962), p. 143.
54. P. Stocks, Lung cancer death rates and content of air of 3,4-benzpyrene in communities near Liverpool (table). *Chemical Carcinogenesis and Cancer,* ed. W. C. Hueper and W. D. Conway (Springfield, Ill.: C. C. Thomas, 1964), p. 124.

55. M. Kuschner, The J. Burns Amberson Lecture: The causes of lung cancer. *American Review of Respiratory Disease* 98, 573-90 (1968).
56. T. Gordon and C. C. Gorst, *Coronary Heart Disease in Adults, United States–1960–1962,* U.S. Department of Health, Education and Welfare, National Center for Health Statistics, P.H.S. Publication 1000, Series 11, No. 10 (Washington, D.C.: U.S. Government Printing Office, 1965).
57. J. N. Morris, *Uses of Epidemiology* (Baltimore: Williams & Wilkins, 1964), pp. 241-43.
58. R. Schiffman and E. Landau, Use of indexes of air pollution potential in mortality studies. *Journal of the Air Pollution Control Association* 11, 384-86 (1961).
59. R. A. Prindle, Some considerations in the interpretation of air pollution health effects data. *Journal of the Air Pollution Control Association,* 9, 12-21 (1959).
60. N. E. Manos and G. F. Fisher, An index of air pollution and its relation to health. *Journal of the Air Pollution Control Association* 9, 5-11 (1959).
61. N. E. Manos, *Comparative Mortality Among Metropolitan Areas of the United States, 1949–1951,* Public Health Service, Division of Special Health Services, P.H.S. Publication No. 562 (Washington, D.C.: U.S. Government Printing Office, 1957).
62. P. E. Enterline, A. E. Rikli, H. I. Sauer, and M. Hyman, Death rates for coronary heart disease in metropolitan and other areas. *Public Health Reports* 75, 759-66 (1960).
63. H. I. Sauer, Epidemiology of cardiovascular mortality–geographic and ethnic. *American Journal of Public Health* 52, 94-105 (1962).
64. H. C. Chase, Variations in heart disease mortality among counties of New York state. *Public Health Reports* 78, 525-34 (1963).
65. H. A. Tyroler and J. Cassel, Health consequences of culture change: II. The effect of urbanization on coronary heart mortality in rural residents. *Journal of Chronic Diseases* 17, 167-77 (1964).
66. S. L. Syme, M. M. Hyman, and P. E. Enterline, Some social and cultural factors associated with the occurrence of coronary heart disease. *Journal of Chronic Diseases* 17, 277-89 (1964).
67. H. I. Sauer, Epidemiology of cardiovascular mortality–geographic and ethnic. *American Journal of Public Health* 52, 94-105 (1962).
68. S. I. Cohen, M, Deane, and J. R. Goldsmith, Carbon monoxide and survival from myocardial infarction. *Archives of Environmental Health* 19, 510-17 (1969).
69. L. D. Zeidberg, R. J. M. Horton, and E. Landau, The Nashville air pollution study: VI. Cardiovascular disease mortality in relation to air pollution. *Archives of Environmental Health* 15, 225-36 (1967).
70. A. Keys, Coronary heart disease in seven countries. American Heart

Association Monograph, No. 29, *Circulation* 41 (Suppl. Nos. I-1 through I-211) (April, 1970).

71. F. H. Epstein, Coronary heart disease epidemiology revisited. *Circulation* 48, 185-94 (1973).
72. F. W. Stitt, D. G. Clayton, M. D. Crawford, and J. N. Morris, Clinical and biochemical indicators of cardiovascular disease among men living in hard and soft water areas. *Lancet* 1, 122-26 (1973).
73. J. R. Goldsmith, Carbon monoxide and coronary heart disease (Editorial). *Annals of Internal Medicine* 71, 199-201 (1969).
74. A. C. Hexter and J. R. Goldsmith, Carbon monoxide: Association of community air pollution with mortality. *Science* 172, 265-67 (1971).
75. L. D. Ziedberg, R. J. M. Horton, and E. Landau, Nashville air pollution study: VI. Cardiovascular disease mortality in relation to air pollution. *Archives of Environmental Health* 15, 225-48 (1967).
76. J. R. Goldsmith, Carbon monoxide research–recent and remote. *Archives of Environmental Health* 21, 118-20 (1970).
77. U.S. Department of Health, Education and Welfare, Public Health Service, *The Health Consequences of Smoking, A Report to the Surgeon General: 1971,* DHEW Publication No. (HSM) 71-7513.
78. G. D. Friedman, Cigarette smoking and geographic variation in coronary heart disease mortality in the United States. *Journal of Chronic Diseases* 20, 769-79 (1967).
79. J. R. Goldsmith and S. A. Landaw, Carbon monoxide and human health. *Science* 162, 1352-59 (1968).
80. U.S. Department of Health, Education and Welfare, Public Health Service, Environmental Health Service, *Air Quality Criteria for Carbon Monoxide,* National Air Pollution Control Administration, Publication No. AP-62 (Washington, D.C.: U.S. Government Printing Office, March, 1970), pp. 8-24–8-34.
81. D. A. DeBias, C. M. Banerjee, N. C. Birkhead, W. V. Harper, and L. A. Kazal, Carbon monoxide inhalation effects following myocardial infarction in monkeys. *Archives of Environmental Health* 27, 161-67 (1973).
82. E. Asmussen, Concluding remarks to: A comparison of prolonged exposure to carbon monoxide and hypoxia in man. *Journal of Clinical Investigation* (Suppl. 103) 22, 68-71 (1968).
83. P. J. Lawther and B. T. Commins, Cigarette smoking and exposure to carbon monoxide. *Annals of the New York Academy of Sciences* 174 Art. 1, 135-47 (1970).
84. P. Astrup, K. Kjeldsen, and J. Wanstrup, Effects of carbon monoxide exposure on the arterial walls. *Annals of the New York Academy of Sciences* 174 Art. 1, 294-300 (1970).
85. P. K. Mueller and M. Hitchcock, Air quality criteria: Toxicological appraisal for oxidants, nitrogen oxides, and hydrocarbons. *Journal of the Air Pollution Control Association* 19, 670-76 (1969).

86. S. H. Mudd, F. Irreverre, and L. Laster, Sulfite oxidase deficiency in man: Demonstration of the enzymatic defect. *Science* 156, 1599-1602 (1967).
87. R. Dubos, *Man Adapting* (New Haven: Yale University Press, 1965), pp. 214-15.
88. A. B. Hill, The environment and disease: Association or causation? *Proceedings of the Royal Society of Medicine* 58, 295-300 (1965).
89. B. W. Carnow and P. Meier, Air pollution and pulmonary cancer. *Archives of Environmental Health* 27, 207-18 (September, 1973).
90. G. B. Morgan, G. Ozolins, and E. C. Tabor, Air pollution surveillance systems. *Science* 170, 289-96 (1970).
91. Environmental Protection Agency, *The Economics of Clean Air,* Annual Report of The Administrator to the Congress of the United States (Washington, D.C.: U.S. Government Printing Office, March 1972).
92. A. C. Stern (ed.), *Air Pollution* (3 vols.), 2nd ed. (New York: Academic Press, 1968).
93. M. Eisenbud, Environmental protection in the City of New York. *Science* 170, 706-12 (1970).
94. W. E. Westman and R. M. Gifford, Environmental impact: Controlling the overall level. *Science* 181, 819-25 (1973).
95. L. B. Lave and E. P. Seskin, Air pollution and human health. *Science* 169, 723-33 (1970).
96. L. B. Lave and E. P. Seskin, An analysis of the association between U.S. mortality and air pollution. *Journal of the American Statistical Association* 68, 284-90 (1973).
97. S. S. Epstein, Environmental pathology: A review. *American Journal of Pathology* 66, 352-73 (1972).

CHAPTER 2

1. R. Dunglison, *Human Health* (Philadelphia: Lea & Blanchard, 1844), p. 114.
2. *Ibid.,* p. 112.
3. M. Lerner and O. W. Anderson, *Health Progress in the United States 1900–1960* (Chicago: University of Chicago Press, 1963).
4. H. Zinsser, *Rats, Lice and History* (New York: Bantam Books, 1935), p. 113.
5. S. Smith, The history of public health, 1871–1921, in *A Half Century of Public Health,* ed. M. P. Ravenel (New York: American Public Health Association, 1921), pp. 1-12.
6. J. Snow, *Snow on Cholera: Being A Reprint of Two Papers* (New

York: Hafner Publishing Co., 1965) (originally published, 1849-1855).

7. S. Smith, *The City That Was* (New York: Frank Allaben, 1911).
8. Smith, The history of public health, 1871–1971, pp. 9-10.
9. F. M. Todd, *Eradicating Plague from San Francisco: Report of the Citizens Health Committee* (San Francisco: C. A. Murdock & Co., 1909).
10. R. Dubos, *Mirage of Health: Utopias, Progress, and Biological Change* (New York: Harper & Brothers, 1959).
11. Society Reports, Joint Meeting of the Maryland Public Health Association, The Medical and Chirurgical Faculty, and The Laennec Society, for the Purpose of Discussing Tuberculosis. *Maryland Medical Journal* 45, 128-35 (1902).
12. W. T. Sedgwick, *Principles of Sanitary Science and the Public Health* (New York: MacMillan, 1902).
13. D. T. Smith, N. F. Conant, and H. P. Willett, *Zinsser Microbiology* 14th ed. (New York: Appleton-Century-Crofts, 1968), pp. 697-98.
14. In the three years 1969-1971 there were 1,379 deaths attributed to syphilis in the United States. Crude death rates by residence were 0.3 per 100,000 for metropolitan counties with central cities, 0.1 for suburban counties, and 0.2 for non-metropolitan counties. The number of deaths was too small to permit calculation of the age-adjusted rates shown in figures throughout the text.
15. A. M. Lowell, L. B. Edwards, and C. E. Palmer, *Tuberculosis* (Cambridge, Mass.: Harvard University Press, 1969), p. 79.
16. Dubos, *Mirage of Health: Utopias, Progress, and Biological Change,* pp. 160-162.
17. Lowell, Edwards, and Palmer, *Tuberculosis,* pp. 140-152.
18. F. van der Kuyp, *Tuberculosis Control, Cuyahoga County, 1969* (Sunny Acres Hospital and Cuyahoga County Tuberculosis Clinics, Cleveland, Ohio, 1970).
19. R. A. Vonderlehr and L. J. Usilton, Syphilis among selectees and volunteers. *Journal of the American Medical Association* 117, 1350-51 (1941).
20. T. Gordon and B. Devine, *Findings on the Serologic Test for Syphilis in Adults, United States—1960–1962,* U.S. Department of Health, Education and Welfare, National Center for Health Statistics, P.H.S. Publication No. 1000, Series 11, No. 9 (Washington, D.C.: U.S. Government Printing Office, 1965).
21. C. C. Dauer, R. F. Korns, and L. M. Schuman, *Infectious Diseases* (Cambridge, Mass.: Harvard University Press, 1968), pp. 9-20.
22. W. J. Brown, J. F. Donohue, N. W. Axnick, J. H. Blount, N. H. Ewen, and O. G. Jones, *Syphilis and Other Venereal Diseases* (Cambridge, Mass.: Harvard University Press, 1970).

23. R. L. Meier, The metropolis as a transaction-maximizing system. *Daedalus* 97, 1292-1313 (1968).
24. Dauer, Korns, and Schuman, *Infectious Diseases,* pp. 27, 81.
25. *Ibid.,* pp. 133-38.
26. C. S. Wilder, *Health Characteristics by Geographic Region, Large Metropolitan Areas, and Other Places of Residence, United States—July 1963–June 1965,* U.S. Department of Health, Education and Welfare, National Center for Health Statistics, P.H.S. Publication, No. 1000, Series 10, No. 36 (Washington, D.C.: U.S. Government Printing Office, 1967).
27. Lerner and Anderson, *Health Progress in United States,* pp. 41-53.
28. World Health Organization, WHO Expert Committee on Smallpox Eradication, *Second Report* (World Health Organization Technical Report Series, No. 493), 1972.
29. Dubos, *Mirage of Health: Utopias, Progress, Biological Change.*
30. A. D. Langmuir, Evolution of the concept of surveillance in the United States. *Proceedings of the Royal Society of Medicine* 64, 681-84 (1971).
31. J. R. Quinn (ed.), *Medicine and Public Health in the People's Republic of China,* DHEW Publication No. (NIH) 72-67, U.S. Department of Health, Education and Welfare, Public Health Service (Bethesda, Maryland: National Institutes of Health, 1972.)
32. V. Navarro, Health services in Cuba. *New England Journal of Medicine,* 287, 954-59 (1972).
33. L. Gordis, Effectiveness of comprehensive-care programs in preventing rheumatic fever. *New England Journal of Medicine* 289, 331-35 (1973).
34. E. Barrett-Connor, The epidemiology and control of gonorrhea and syphilis: A reappraisal. *Preventive Medicine* 3, 102-21 (1974).
35. F. M. Burnet, *Natural History of Infectious Disease,* 3rd ed. (Cambridge: Cambridge University Press, 1962), p. ix.

CHAPTER 3

1. R. Hofstadter, *The Age of Reform* (New York: Random House, 1955), p. 23.
2. D. Hunter, *The Diseases of Occupations,* 4th ed. (Boston: Little, Brown, 1969), pp. 90-146.
3. C. A. D'Alonzo, History of industrial medicine, in *Modern Occupational Medicine,* eds. A. J. Fleming, C. A. D'Alonzo, and J. A. Zapp (Philadelphia: Lea & Febiger, 1960), p. 20-27.
4. Factory Inspectors of the State of New York, *First Annual Report* (Albany: The Argus Company, 1887).

5. J. Riis, *How the Other Half Lives* (New York: Hill and Wang, 1957) (originally published in 1890) pp. 92, 178.
6. U.S. Congress, Senate, *Report on Conditions of Employment in Iron and Steel Industry,* 62nd Cong., 2nd sess., 1912, S. 301, pp. 8-10.
7. A. Hamilton, *Exploring the Dangerous Trades: The Autobiography* (Boston: Little, Brown, 1943), pp. 3-17.
8. C. A. D'Alonzo, History of industrial medicine, in *Modern Occupational Medicine,* eds. A. J. Fleming, C. A. D'Alonzo, and J. A. Zapp (Philadelphia: Lea & Febiger, 1960), p. 24.
9. U.S. Department of Commerce, Bureau of the Census, *Statistical Abstract of the United States, 1972,* 93rd ed. (Washington, D.C.: U.S. Government Printing Office, 1972), Table 383.
10. U.S. Department of Commerce, Bureau of the Census, *Historical Statistics of the United States, Colonial Times to 1957: A Statistical Abstract Supplement* (Washington, D.C.: U.S. Government Printing, Office, 1960), Table D785-792.
11. W. I. Trattner, *Crusade for the Children: A History of the National Child Labor Committee and Child Labor Reform in America* (Chicago: Quadrangle Books, 1970), pp. 226-29.
12. G. A. Ryan, Injuries in urban and rural traffic accidents: A comparison of two studies, *Proceeding of Eleventh Stapp Car Crash Conference, 1967,* Society of Automotive Engineers, Inc., Two Pennsylvania Plaza (New York, 1969), pp. 479-88.
13. G. V. Graham, *Persons Injured and Disability Days due to Injury, United States–July 1965–June 1967,* U.S. Department of Health, Education and Welfare, National Center for Health Statistics, P.H.S. Publication No. 1000, Series 10, No. 58 (Washington, D.C.: U.S. Government Printing Office, 1970).
14. C. S. Wilder, *Type of Injuries, Incidence and Associated Disability, United States–July 1965–June 1967,* U.S. Department of Health, Education and Welfare, National Center for Health Statistics, P.H.S. Publication No. 1000, Series 10, No. 57 (Washington, D.C.: U.S. Government Printing Office, 1969).
15. U.S. Department of Commerce, Bureau of the Census, *Statistical Abstract of the United States,* 1972, 93rd ed. (Washington, D.C.: U.S. Government Printing Office, 1972), Table 383.
16. C. H. Brooks, *Work Injuries Among Blue-collar Workers and Disability Days, United States, July 1966–June 1967,* U.S. Department of Health, Education and Welfare, National Center for Health Statistics, Vital and Health Statistics, Series 10, No. 68, DHEW Publication No. (HSM) 72-1035 (Washington, D.C.: U.S. Government Printing Office, 1972).
17. U.S. Department of Health, Education and Welfare, Public Health Service, National Institute for Occupational Safety and Health, *The*

Toxic Substances List, 1973 Edition (Washington, D.C.: U.S. Government Printing Office, 1973).

18. L. A. Sagan, Human Costs of Nuclear Power. *Science* 177, 487-93 (1972).
19. Special Task Force, *Work in America: Report of a Special Task Force to the Secretary of Health, Education and Welfare* (Cambridge, Mass.: MIT Press, 1973).
20. A. W. Kornhauser, *Mental Health of the Industrial Worker: A Detroit Study* (New York: Wiley, 1965).
21. C. S. Wilder, *Time Lost from Work among the Currently Employed Population, United States–1968,* U.S. Department of Health, Education and Welfare, National Center for Health Statistics, Vital and Health Statistics, Series 10, No. 71 (Washington, D.C.: Government Printing Office, 1972).
22. U.S. Department of Commerce, Bureau of the Census, *Statistical Abstract of the United States, 1974,* 95th ed. (Washington, D.C.: U.S. Government Printing Office, 1974), Table 559.
23. C. S. Wilder, *Health Characteristics by Geographic Region, Large Metropolitan Areas, and Other Places of Residence, United States–July 1963–June 1965,* U.S. Department of Health, Education and Welfare, National Center for Health Statistics, P.H.S. Publication No. 1000, Series 10, No. 36 (Washington, D.C.: U.S. Government Printing Office, 1967).
24. G. A. Gleeson, *Age Patterns in Medical Care, Illness, and Disability, United States–July 1963–June 1965,* U.S. Department of Health, Education and Welfare, National Center for Health Statistics, P.H.S. Publication No. 1000, Series 10, No. 32 (Washington, D.C.: U.S. Government Printing Office, 1966).
25. A. L. Jackson, *Children and Youth: Selected Health Characteristics–United States, 1958 and 1968,* U.S. Department of Health, Education and Welfare, National Center for Health Statistics, P.H.S. Publication No. 1000, Series 10, No. 62 (Washington, D.C.: U.S. Government Printing Office, 1971).
26. C. S. Wilder, *Limitation of Activity and Mobility Due to Chronic Conditions, United States–July 1965–June 1966,* U.S. Department of Health, Education and Welfare, National Center for Health Statistics, P.H.S. Publication No. 1000, Series 10, No. 45 (Washington, D.C.: U.S. Government Printing Office, 1968).
27. G. Sparer and L. M. Okada, Chronic conditions and physical use patterns in ten urban poverty areas. *Medical Care* 12, 549-60 (1974).
28. J. N. Cross, *Guide to the Community Control of Alcoholism* (New York: American Public Health Association, 1968).
29. D. Cahalan and I. H. Cisin, American drinking practices: Summary of findings from a national probability sample. *Quarterly Journal Studies*

on Alcohol 29 (1968): Part I. Extent of drinking by population subgroups, 130-51; Part II. Measurement of massed versus spaced drinking, 642-56.

30. D. J. Myerson, A three-year study of a group of skid row alcoholics, *Alcoholism: Basic Aspects and Treatment,* ed. H. E. Himwich (Washington, D.C.: American Association for the Advancement of Science, 1957), pp. 151-62.
31. J. C. Ball, D. M. Englander, and C. D. Chambers, The incidence and prevalence of opiate addiction in the United States, in *The Epidemiology of Opiate Addiction in the United States,* eds, J. C. Ball and C. D. Chambers (Springfield, Ill.: C. C. Thomas, 1970), Chapter 1.
32. *Ibid.,* pp. 68-78.
33. R. L. DuPont, Profile of a heroin-addiction epidemic. *New England Journal of Medicine* 285, 320-24 (1971).
34. P. H. Hughes, N. W. Barker, G. A. Crawford, and J. H. Jaffe, The natural history of a heroin epidemic. *American Journal of Public Health* 62, 995-1001 (1972).
35. J. W. Spelman, Heroin addiction: The epidemics of the '70's. *Archives of Environmental Health* 21, 589-90 (1970).
36. M. Helpern, Fatalities from narcotic addiction in New York City. Incidence, circumstances, and pathologic findings. *Human Pathology* 3, 13-21 (1972).
37. J. C. Ball, D. M. Englander, and C. D. Chambers, The incidence and prevalence of opiate addiction in the United States, in *The Epidemiology of Opiate Addiction in the United States,* ed. J. C. Ball and C. D. Chambers (Springfield, Ill.: C. C. Thomas, 1970), p. 76.
38. A. W. McCoy, *The Politics of Heroin in Southeast Asia* (New York: Harper & Row, 1972).
39. U.S. Task Force on Narcotics and Drug Abuse, *Task Force Report: Narcotics and Drug Abuse* (Washington, D.C.: U.S. Government Printing Office, 1967).
40. J. Peel and M. Potts, *Textbook of Contraceptive Practice* (Cambridge, Mass.: Cambridge University Press, 1969), pp. 206-8.
41. W. J. Curran, The abortion decisions: The Supreme Court as moralist, scientist, historian and legislator. *New England Journal of Medicine* 288, 950-51 (1973).
42. J. Blake, Abortion and public opinion: The 1960–1970 decade. *Science* 171, 540-55 (1971).
43. S. Shapiro, E. R. Schlesinger, and R. E. L. Nesbitt, Jr., *Infant, Perinatal, Maternal, and Childhood Morality in the United States* (Cambridge, Mass.: Harvard University Press, 1968), pp. 153-54; Appendix Table II. 4a.
44. J. Pakter, D. O'Hare, F. Nelson, and M. Svigir, Two years experience in New York City with the liberalized abortion law–progress and problems. *American Journal of Public Health* 63, 524-35 (1973).

45. A. J. Clague and S. J. Ventura, *Trends in Illegitimacy, United States—1940–1965,* U.S. Department of Health, Education and Welfare, National Center for Health Statistics, P.H.S. Publication No. 1000, Series 21, No. 15 (Washington, D.C.: U.S. Government Printing Office, 1968).
46. R. L. Heuser, S. J. Ventura, and F. H. Godley, *Natality Statistics Analysis, United States, 1965–1967,* U.S. Department of Health, Education and Welfare, National Center for Health Statistics, P.H.S. Publication No. 1000, Series 21, No. 19 (Washington, D.C.: U.S. Government Printing Office, 1970).
47. J. Sklar and B. Berkov, The effects of legal abortion on legitimate and illegitimate birth rates: The California experience. *Studies in Family Planning* 4, 281-92 (1973).
48. U.S. Department of Commerce, Bureau of the Census, Current Population Reports, *Trends in Social and Economic Conditions in Metropolitan and Non-metropolitan Areas,* Series P-23, No. 33 (Washington, D.C.: U.S. Government Printing Office, 1970).
49. E. Durkheim, *Suicide: A Study in Sociology* (Glencoe, Ill.: Free Press, 1962) (originally published in 1897).
50. H. Harlan, Five hundred homicides. *Journal of Criminal Law, Criminology and Police Science* 40, 736-52 (1949-50).
51. H. A. Bullock, Urban homicide in theory and fact. *Journal of Criminal Law, Criminology and Police Science* 45, 565-75 (1954-55).
52. M. E. Wolfgang, *Patterns in Criminal Homicide* (Philadelphia: University of Pennsylvania Press, 1958).
53. R. C. Bensing and O. Schroeder, Jr., *Homicide in an Urban Community* (Springfield, Ill.: C. C. Thomas, 1960).
54. C. S. Hirsch, N. B. Rushforth, A. B. Ford, and L. Adelson, Homicide and suicide in a metropolitan county: 1. Long-term trends. *Journal of the American Medical Association* 223, 900-5 (1973).
55. R. Langberg, *Homicide in the United States,* U.S. Department of Health, Education and Welfare, National Center for Health Statistics, Vital and Health Statistics, Series 20, no. 6 (Washington, D.C.: U.S. Government Printing Office, 1967), pp. 1-33.
56. T. F. Pettigrew and R. B. Spier, The ecological structure of Negro homicide. *American Journal of Sociology* 67, 621-29 (1962).
57. M. E. Wolfgang, *Patterns in Criminal Homicide,* (Philadelphia: University of Pennsylvania Press, 1958), p. 331.
58. F. P. Graham, A Contemporary History of American Crime, in *Violence in America: Historical and Comparative Perspectives,* eds. H. D. Graham and T. R. Gurr (New York: The New American Library, 1969), p. 78.
59. C. Tilly, Race and migration to the American city, in *The Metropolitan Enigma: Inquiries into the Nature and Dimensions of America's*

Urban Crisis, ed. J. Q. Wilson (Cambridge, Mass.: Harvard University Press, 1968), pp. 135-57.
60. M. E. Wolfgang, Urban crime, in *The Metropolitan Enigma,* ed. J. Q. Wilson (Cambridge, Mass.: Harvard University Press, 1968), pp. 245-81.
61. N. B. Rushforth, C. S. Hirsch, A. B. Ford, and L. Adelson, Accidental firearms fatalities in a metropolitan county (1958–1973). *American Journal of Epidemiology* 100, 499-505 (1974).
62. R. Ellison, *Shadow and Act* (New York: Random House, 1964), pp. 295-96.
63. L. Bergner and A. S. Yerby, Low income and barriers to use of health services. *New England Journal of Medicine* 278, 541-46 (1968).
64. S. J. Ventura, S. M. Taffel, and E. Spratley, Vital and Health Statistics for Low-Income Areas in 19 Large Cities, 1969–1971 (Paper presented at annual meeting, American Public Health Association, New Orleans, Louisiana, October 24, 1974.)
65. J. B. Calhoun, Population density and social pathology, in *The Urban Condition: People and Policy in the Metropolis* ed. L. J. Duhl (New York: Simon and Schuster, 1969), pp. 33-43.
66. D. A. Hamburg, Crowding, stranger contact, and aggressive behaviour, *Society Stress and Disease, Vol. 1 The Psychosocial Environment and Psychosomatic Diseases,* ed. L. Levi (London: Oxford University Press, 1971), pp. 209-18.
67. *New York Times,* Negro migration to North found steady since '40's, 4 March 1971.
68. P. F. Drucker, Worker and work in the metropolis. *Daedalus* 97, 1243-76 (1968).
69. D. P. Moynihan, Poverty in Cities, in *The Metropolitan Enigma,* ed. J. Q. Wilson (Cambridge, Mass.: Harvard University Press, 1968), pp. 335-49.
70. National Commission on the Causes and Prevention of Violence, *To Establish Justice, To Insure Domestic Tranquility: Final Report* (Washington, D.C.: U.S. Government Printing Office, 1969).
71. U.S. Department of Health, Education and Welfare, *Human Investment Programs: Delivery of Health Services for the Poor* (Washington, D.C.: U.S. Government Printing Office, 1968).
72. P. V. V. Hamill, F. E. Johnston, and S. Lemeshow, *Height and Weight of Children: Socioeconomic Status,* U.S. Department of Health, Education and Welfare, National Center for Health Statistics, DHEW Publication No. (HSM) 73-1601, Series 11, No. 119 (Washington, D.C.: U.S. Government Printing Office, 1972).
73. O. Lewis, *La Vida: A Puerto Rican Family in the Culture of Poverty—San Juan and New York* (New York: Random House, 1965) pp. xlii-lii.
74. E. J. Ryan, Personal identity in an urban slum, in *The Urban Con-*

dition: People and Policy in the metropolis, ed. L. J. Duhl (New York: Simon and Schuster, 1969), pp. 135-50.

75. P. Brodeur, Annals of Industry (Casualties of the Workplace–I). *New Yorker* 29 October, 1973, 44ff.
76. S. S. Epstein, Environmental pathology: A review. *American Journal of Pathology* 66, 352-73 (1972).
77. J. Gooding, *The Job Revolution* (New York: Walker and Co., 1972), pp. 91-108.
78. Institute of Medicine, Panel on Health Services Research, Infant death: An analysis by maternal risk and health care, *Contrasts in Health Status,* Vol. 1 (Washington, D.C.: National Academy of Sciences, 1973).
79. P. Marris, A report on urban renewal in the United States, in *The Urban Condition: People and Policy in the Metropolis,* ed. L. J. Duhl (New York: Simon and Schuster, 1969), pp. 113-34.
80. A. B. Shostak, The future of poverty, in *Poverty and Health: A Sociological Analysis,* eds. J. Kosa, A. Antonovsky, and I. K. Zola (Cambridge, Mass.: Commonwealth Fund Harvard University Press, 1969), pp. 274-79.
81. D. P. Moynihan, *Maximum Feasible Misunderstanding: Community Action in the War on Poverty* (New York: The Free Press, 1970).
82. C. L. Schultze, E. R. Fried, A. M. Rivlin, and N. H. Teeters, *Setting National Priorities: The 1972 Budget* (Washington, D.C.: The Brookings Institution, 1971).
83. H. George, *Progress and Poverty* (New York: Doubleday & McClure, 1879), p. 9.
84. P. Barnes, The GNP machine: How wealth is distributed. *New Republic* (30 September 1972), pp. 18-20.

CHAPTER 4

1. Case from the files of University Hospitals of Cleveland and private records. The name and some details have been changed.
2. C. F. Westoff, The populations of the developed countries. *Scientific American* 231 (3), 109-20 (September 1974).
3. C. S. Wilder, *Chronic Conditions and Limitations of Activity and Mobility, United States–July 1965–June 1967,* U.S. Department of Health, Education and Welfare, National Center for Health Statistics, P.H.S. Publication No. 1000, Series 10, No. 61 (Washington, D.C.: U.S. Government Printing Office, 1971).
4. C. S. Wilder, *Limitation of Activity Due to Chronic Conditions, United States, 1969 and 1970,* U.S. Department of Health, Education and Welfare, National Center for Health Statistics, DHEW Publication

No. (HSM) 73-1506, Series 10, No. 80 (Washington, D.C.: Government Printing Office, 1973).

5. G. Sparer and A. Alderman, Data needs for planning neighborhood health centers. *American Journal of Public Health* 61, 796-806 (1971).
6. E. Cumming and W. E. Henry, *Growing Old: The Process of Disengagement* (New York: Basic Books, 1961).
7. A. Downs, Who are the urban poor?, Committee for Economic Development, Supplementary Paper (New York: Committee for Economic Development, 1968).
8. J. A. Pechman, H. J. Aaron, and M. K. Taussig, *Social Security: Perspectives for Reform* (Washington, D.C.: The Brookings Institution, 1968), pp. 17-26.
9. L. A. Epstein and J. H. Murray, *The Aged Population of the United States: The 1963 Social Security Survey of the Aged,* U.S. Department of Health, Education and Welfare, Social Security Administration Office of Research and Statistics, Research Report No. 19 (Washington, D.C.: U.S. Government Printing Office, 1967).
10. *Ibid.,* p. 420.
11. U.S. Congress, Senate, Special Committee on Aging, *Developments in Aging, 1969,* 91st Cong., 2nd Sess., 1970, Rept. 91-875, pp. 91-101.
12. E. Shanas, P. Townsend, D. Wedderburn, H. Friis, P. Milhj, and J. Stehouwer (New York: Atherton Press, 1968), Table II-1.
13. M. H. Wilder, *Home Care for Persons 55 Years and Over, July 1966–June 1968,* U.S. Department of Health, Education and Welfare, National Center for Health Statistics, DHEW Publication No. (HSM) 72-1062 (Washington, D.C.: U.S. Government Printing Office, 1972).
14. J. W. Davis and M. J. Gibbin, An areawide examination of nursing home use, misuse and nonuse. *American Journal of Public Health* 61, 1146-55 (1971).
15. U.S. Congress, Senate, Special Committee on Aging, *Developments in Aging,* 1969, 91st Cong., 2nd Sess., 1970, Rept. 91-875, p. 35.
16. M. Blenkner, M. Bloom, and M. Nielsen, A research and demonstration project of protective services. *Social Casework* 52, 483-99 (1971).
17. L. Srole, T. S. Langner, S. T. Michael, M. K. Opler, and T. A. C. Rennie, *Mental Health in the Metropolis: The Midtown Manhattan Study* (New York: Blakiston-McGraw-Hill Book Co., 1962), vol. 1, pp. 159-62, 218-22, 346.
18. E. M. Gruenberg, A review of *Mental Health in the Metropolis: The Midtown Manhattan Study. Milbank Memorial Fund Quarterly* 41, 77-94 (1963).
19. Pechman, Aaron, and Taussig, *Social Security: Perspectives for Reform,* p. 8.
20. M. Lerner and O. W. Anderson, *Health Progress in the United States 1900–1960* (Chicago: University of Chicago Press, 1963), p. 110.

21. E. G. Jaco, *The Social Epidemiology of Mental Disorders* (New York: Russell Sage Foundation, 1960), p. 93.
22. Srole, Langner, Michael, Opler, and Rennie, *Mental Health in Metropolis: The Midtown Manhattan Study,* pp. 271-72.
23. T. F. Pugh and B. MacMahon, *Epidemiologic Findings in United States Mental Hospital Data* (Boston: Little, Brown, 1962), pp. 30-37.
24. C. Tilly, Race and migration to the American city, in *The Metropolitan Enigma: Inquiries into the Nature and Dimensions of America's "Urban Crisis,"* ed. J. Q. Wilson (Cambridge, Mass.: Harvard University Press, 1968), pp. 135-57.
25. T. Wan, Social differentials in selected work-limiting chronic conditions. *Journal of Chronic Diseases* 25, 365-74 (1972).
26. M. Fried, Social differences in mental health, in *Poverty and Health: A Sociological Analysis,* eds. J. Kosa, A. Antonovsky, and I. K. Zola (Cambridge, Mass.: Harvard University Press, 1969), pp. 113-167.
27. A. G. Dingfelder, *Chronic Conditions Causing Activity Limitation, United States–July 1963–June 1965,* U.S. Department of Health, Education and Welfare, National Center for Health Statistics, P.H.S. Publication No. 1000, Series 10, No. 51 (Washington, D.C.: U.S. Government Printing Office, 1969).
28. H. J. Dupuy, A. Engel, B. K. Devine, J. Scanlon, and L. Querec, *Selected Symptoms of Psychological Distress, United States,* U.S. Department of Health, Education and Welfare, National Center for Health Statistics, P.H.S. Publication No. 1000, Series 11, No. 37 (Washington, D.C.: U.S. Government Printing Office, 1970).
29. O. Lewis, *La Vida: A Puerto Rican Family in the Culture of Poverty –San Juan and New York* (New York: Vintage Books Random House, 1965), pp. xlii-lii.
30. H. Blumenfeld, Transportation in the modern metropolis, in *Internal Structure of the City: Readings on Space and Environment,* ed. L. S. Bourne (New York: Oxford University Press, 1971), pp. 231-39.
31. J. R. Meyer, Urban transportation, in *The Metropolitan Enigma,* ed. J. Q. Wilson (Cambridge, Mass.: Harvard University Press, 1968), pp. 42-69.
32. J. G. Wofford, Transportation, in *The State and the Poor,* eds. S. H. Beer and R. E. Barringer (Cambridge, Mass.: Winthrop Publishers, 1970), pp. 166-92.
33. O. Newman, *Defensible Space: Crime Prevention through Urban Design* (New York: MacMillan, 1972).
34. B. J. Frieden, Housing: Creating the supply, in *The State and the Poor,* eds. S. H. Beer and R. E. Barringer (Cambridge, Mass.: Winthrop Publishers, 1970), pp. 106-34.
35. J. Jacobs, *The Death and Life of Great American Cities* (New York: Random House, 1961), pp. 392-404.

36. Anonymous, Homing in on housing. *Architectural Forum* (November, 1972), pp. 42-51.
37. White House Conference on Aging, 1971, *Toward A National Policy on Aging,* vol. 2 (Washington, D.C.: U.S. Government Printing Office, 1973), pp. 29-36.
38. M. A. Mendelson, *Tender Loving Greed* (New York: Knopf, 1974).
39. A. B. Nelson, *Prevalence of Chronic Conditions and Impairments among Residents of Nursing and Personal Care Homes May-June 1964,* U.S. Department of Health, Education and Welfare, National Center for Health Statistics, P.H.S. Publication No. 1000, Series 12, No. 8 (Washington, D.C.: U.S. Government Printing Office, 1967).
40. J. A. Solon, Medical care: Its social and organizational aspects: Nursing homes and medical care. *New England Journal of Medicine* 269, 1067-74 (1963).
41. S. Levey, H. S. Ruchlin, B. A. Stotsky, D. R. Kinloch, and W. Oppenheim, An appraisal of nursing home care. *Journal of Gerontology* 28, 222-28 (1973).
42. J. Zusman, Development of the social breakdown syndrome concept, in *Evaluating the Effectiveness of Community Mental Health Services,* ed. E. M. Gruenberg (New York: Milbank Memorial Fund, 1966), pp. 363-94.
43. W. W. Jepson, Metropolitan mental health center development, in *The Practice of Community Mental Health,* ed. H. Grunebaum (Boston: Little, Brown, 1970), pp. 439-67.
44. P. C. Talkington, Critical issues in psychiatry: A call for a reassessment of our nation's mental health care. *Hospital and Community Psychiatry* 24, 17-22 (1973).
45. Pechman, Aaron, and Taussig, *Social Security: Perspectives for Reform,* p. 1.
46. *Ibid.,* p. 105.
47. *Ibid.,* pp. 214-27.
48. U.S. Congress, Senate, Special Committee on Aging, *Developments in Aging, 1969,* p. 3.
49. National Assembly for Social Policy and Development, *Policy Statement on Income Maintenance* (New York: NASPD, 1972).
50. C. I. Schottland, *The Social Security Program in the United States,* 2nd ed. (New York: Appleton-Century-Crofts, 1970).
51. Pechman, Aaron, and Taussig, *Social Security: Perspectives for Reform.*
52. H. M. Somers and A. R. Somers, *Medicare and the Hospitals: Issues and Prospects* (Washington, D.C.: The Brookings Institution, 1967).
53. S. E. Bernard and E. Feingold, The impact of Medicaid. *Wisconsin Law Review,* 726-55 (1970).
54. R. C. Rorem, The economics of health care, in *Depth and Extent of the Geriatic Problem,* ed. M. Field (Springfield, Ill.: C. C. Thomas, 1970), pp. 63-76.

55. U.S. Code, *Congressional and Administrative News,* 93rd Cong., 1st Sess., 1973, 1: 38-79; 1327-61.
56. Shanas, *Old People in Three Industrial Societies,* Table IV, p. 8.
57. *Ibid.,* pp. 18-48.
58. *Ibid.,* pp. 18-19.
59. S. Clavan and E. Vatter, The affiliated family: A device for integrating old and young. *Gerontologist* 12, 407-12 (1972).
60. N. B. Ryder, The family in developed countries. *Scientific American* 231, 122-32 (1974).

CHAPTER 5

1. E. Jarvis, On the supposed increase of insanity. *American Journal of Insanity* 8, 333-64 (1852).
2. K. B. Sohler and J. D. Thompson, Jarvis' Law and the planning of mental health services. *Public Health Report* 85, 503-15 (1970).
3. M. I. Roemer and M. Shain, *Hospital Utilization under Insurance, Hospital Monograph Series No. 6* (Chicago: American Hospital Association, 1959), p. 12.
4. J. G. Anderson, Demographic factors affecting health services utilization: A causal model. *Medical Care* 11, 104-20 (1973).
5. G. W. Shannon, J. L. Skinner, and R. L. Bashshur, Time and distance: The journey for medical care. *International Journal of Health Services* 3, 237-44 (1973).
6. U.S. Department of Health, Education and Welfare, Public Health Service, Bureau of Health Professions Education and Manpower Training, *Health Manpower Source Book,* Section 20, Manpower Supply and Educational Statistics for Selected Health Occupations: 1968, PHS Publication No. 263, Section 20 (Washington, D.C.: U.S. Government Printing Office, 1969), Table 33.
7. U.S. Department of Health, Education and Welfare, Public Health Service, National Center for Health Statistics, *Health Resources Statistics, 1974,* DHEW Publication No. (HRA) 75-1509 (Washington, D.C.: U.S. Government Printing Office, 1974), Table 85.
8. J. L. Dorsey, Physician distribution in Boston and Brookline, 1940 and 1961. *Medical Care* 7, 429-40 (1969).
9. R. L. Bashshur, G. W. Shannon, and C. A. Metzner, The application of three-dimensional analogue models to the distribution of medical care facilities. *Medical Care* 8, 395-407 (1970).
10. Chicago Board of Health, *Medical Care Report* (Chicago: Chicago Board of Health, 1966).
11. U.S. Department of Health, Education and Welfare, Public Health Service, Bureau of Health Professions Education and Manpower Training, *Health Manpower Source Book, Section 20,* Table 47.

12. U.S. Department of Health, Education and Welfare, Division of Dental Health, *Compilation: State Dentist Manpower Reports, 1965-1967* (Washington, D.C.: U.S. Government Printing Office, 1970).
13. A. Donabedian, S. J. Axelrod, C. Swearingen, and J. Jameson, *Medical Care Chart Book,* 5th ed. (Ann Arbor: University of Michigan, 1972), Chart E-3.
14. E. Levine and E. D. Marshall, Nursing manpower, in *Health Manpower, United States, 1965-1967,* U.S. Department of Health, Education and Welfare, National Center for Health Statistics, P.H.S. Publication No. 1000, Series 14, No. 1 (Washington, D.C.: U.S. Government Printing Office, 1968).
15. W. O. Spitzer, The small general hospital: Problems and solutions. *Milbank Memorial Fund Quarterly* 48, 413-47 (1970).
16. R. L. Bashshur, G. W. Shannon, and C. A. Metzner, Some ecological differentials in the use of medical services. *Health Services Research* 6, 61-75 (1971).
17. C. S. Wilder, *Dental Visits: Volume and Interval since Last Visit, United States, 1969,* U.S. Department of Health, Education and Welfare, National Center for Health Statistics, Vital and Health Statistics, Series 10, No. 76, DHEW Publication No. (HSM) 73-1502 (Washington, D.C.: U.S. Government Printing Office, 1972), Table 5.
18. C. S. Wilder, *Physician Visits: Volume and Interval since Last Visit, United States, 1969,* U.S. Department of Health, Education and Welfare, National Center for Health Statistics, Vital and Health Statistics, Series 10, No. 75, DHEW Publication No. (HSM) 73-1064 (Washington, D.C.: U.S. Government Printing Office, 1972), Table 6.
19. *Ibid.,* Table B.
20. T. W. Bice, R. L. Eichhorn, and P. D. Fox, Socioeconomic status and use of physician services: A reconsideration. *Medical Care* 10, 261-71 (1972).
21. G. Sparer and L. M. Okada, Chronic conditions and physician use patterns in ten urban poverty areas. *Medical Care* 12, 549-60 (1974).
22. N. Piore and D. Lewis, Patterns of Hospital Outpatient Use in Fifty Cities of the United States (Paper presented at annual meeting of American Public Health Association, Atlantic City, New Jersey, November 16, 1972).
23. A. V. Hurtado, D. K. Freeborn, J. E. Myers, and M. A. Davis, Unscheduled use of ambulatory care services. *Medical Care* 12, 498-511 (1974).
24. J. A. Roth, The treatment of the sick, in *Poverty and Health: A Sociological Analysis,* eds. J. Kosa, A. Antonovsky, and I. K. Zola (Cambridge, Mass.: Harvard University Press, 1969), pp. 215-43.
25. M. L. Bauer, *Differentials in Health Characteristics by Color, United States–July 1965–June 1967,* U.S. Department of Health, Education

and Welfare, Public Health Service, National Center for Health Statistics, P.H.S. Publication No. 1000, Series 10, No. 56 (Washington, D.C.: U.S. Government Printing Office, 1969).

26. G. A. Gleeson, *Hospital and Surgical Insurance Coverage, United States–1968,* U.S. Department of Health, Education and Welfare, National Center for Health Statistics, Vital and Health Statistics, Series 10, No. 66, DHEW Publication No. (HSM) 72-1033 (Washington, D.C.: U.S. Government Printing Office, 1972).
27. M. Krakowski, M. Werboff, and B. Hoffnar, *Availability and Use of Health Services: Rural-Urban Comparison,* Economic Research Service, U.S. Department of Agriculture, Agricultural Economic Report No. 139 (Washington, D.C.: U.S. Government Printing Office, 1968).
28. World Health Organization, Urban Health Services: Fifth Report of the Expert Committee on Public Health Administration, *Urban Health Services,* W.H.O. Technical Report Series No. 250 (Geneva: World Health Organization, 1963).
29. D. Palmiere, Community health planning, in *Medicine in a Changing Society,* eds. L. Corey, S. E. Saltman, and M. F. Epstein (St. Louis: C. V. Mosby, 1972), pp. 59-82.
30. B. Abel-Smith, Major patterns of financing and organization of medical care in countries other than the United States, in *Medicine in a Changing Society,* eds. L. Corey, S. E. Saltman, and M. F. Epstein (St. Louis: C. V. Mosby, 1972), pp. 211-28.
31. U.S. Department of Health, Education and Welfare, Social Security Administration, *Medical Care Expenditures, Prices, and Costs: Background Book,* DHEW Publication No. (SSA) 74-11909 (Washington, D.C.: U.S. Government Printing Office, 1973).
32. E. W. Saward, The relevance of prepaid group practice to effective delivery of health services, in *Medicine in a Changing Society,* eds. L. Corey, S. E. Saltman, and M. F. Epstein (St. Louis: C. V. Mosby, 1972), pp. 128-37.
33. J. A. Vohs, R. V. Anderson, and R. Straus, Critical issues in HMO strategy. *New England Journal of Medicine* 286, 1082-86 (1972).
34. S. Shapiro, End result measurements of quality of medical care. *Milbank Memorial Fund Quarterly* 45 (Part 2), 7-30 (1967).
35. M. R. Greenlick, D. K. Freeborn, T. J. Colombo, J. A. Prussin, and E. A. Saward, Comparing the use of medical care services by a medically indigent and a general membership population in a comprehensive prepaid group practice program. *Medical Care* 10, 187-200 (1972).
36. M. A. Morehead, R. S. Donaldson, and M. R. Servalli, Comparisons between OEO neighborhood health centers and other health care providers of ratings of the quality of health care. *American Journal of Public Health* 61, 1294-1306 (1971).

37. A. M. Sadler, B. L. Sadler, and A. A. Bliss, *The Physician's Assistant: Today and Tomorrow* (New Haven, Conn.: Yale University Press, 1972).
38. U.S. Department of Health, Education and Welfare, Social Security Administration, *Medical Care Expenditures, Prices, and Costs: Background Book,* DHEW Publication No. (SSA) 74-11909 (Washington, D.C.: U.S. Government Printing Office, 1973), p. 87.
39. R. Andersen, B. Smedby, and O. W. Anderson, *Medical Care Use in Sweden and the United States: A Comparative Analysis of Systems and Behavior* (Chicago: University of Chicago, Center for Health Administration Studies, 1970).
40. J. W. Meigs, Occupation, industrialization, and health, in *Preventive Medicine,* eds. D. W. Clark and B. MacMahon (Boston: Little, Brown, 1967), pp. 677-711.
41. D. W. Clark, Social welfare, in *Preventive Medicine,* eds. D. W. Clark and B. MacMahon (Boston: Little, Brown, 1967), pp. 781-812.
42. P. E. Enterline, V. Salter, A. D. McDonald, and J. C. McDonald, Distribution of medical services before and after "free" medical care: The Quebec experience. *New England Journal of Medicine* 289, 1174-78 (1973).

CHAPTER 6

1. A. M. Lowell, L. B. Edwards, and C. E. Palmer, *Tuberculosis* (Cambridge, Mass.: Harvard University Press, 1969), p. 79.
2. L. B. Edwards and C. E. Palmer, Tuberculous infection, in *Tuberculosis,* eds. A. M. Lowell, L. B. Edwards, and C. E. Palmer (Cambridge, Mass.: Harvard University Press, 1969), p. 146.
3. Cuyahoga County Tuberculosis Clinics, *Tuberculosis Control, Cuyahoga County, 1969* (Cleveland, Ohio: Cuyahoga County Tuberculosis Clinics, 1972).
4. Lowell, Edwards, and Palmer, *Tuberculosis,* pp. 84-93.
5. Edwards and Palmer, Tuberculous infection, in *Tuberculosis,* pp. 176-179.
6. Lowell, Edwards, and Palmer, *Tuberculosis,* pp. 29-30.
7. J. B. Stocklen, M.D., Controller of Chronic Illness and Tuberculosis in Cuyahoga County, Ohio, personal communication.
8. W. B. Beck, Acute appendicitis and incidental appendectomy, in *The Acute Abdomen and Emergent Lesions of the Gastrointestinal Tract,* eds. H. R. Hawthorne, A. S. Frobese, and J. A. Sterling (Springfield, Ill.: C. C. Thomas, 1967), pp. 254-61.
9. K. B. Castleton, C. B. Puestow, and D. Sauer, Is appendicitis decreasing in frequency? *Archives of Surgery* 78, 794-801 (1959).

10. H. W. Green and R. M. Watkins, *Appendicitis in Cleveland, 1946* (mimeo), Cleveland Health Council, 1001 Huron Road, Cleveland, Ohio.
11. S. Shapiro, E. R. Schlesinger, and R. E. L. Nesbitt, Jr., *Infant, Perinatal, Maternal, and Childhood Mortality in the United States* (Cambridge, Mass.: Harvard University Press, 1968), pp. 159-63.
12. *Ibid.,* Preface, pp. v-vii.
13. *Ibid.*, pp. 3-46.
14. H. C. Chase, The position of the United States in international comparisons of health status. *American Journal of Public Health* 62, 581-89 (1972).
15. Chicago Board of Health, *Medical Care Report* (Chicago, Ill.: September, 1966).
16. B. MacMahon, M. G. Kovar, and J. J. Feldman, *Infant Mortality Rates: Socioeconomic Factors,* U.S. Department of Health, Education and Welfare, National Center for Health Statistics, Series 22, No. 14, DHEW Publication No. (HMS) 72-1045 (Washington, D.C.: U.S. Government Printing Office, 1972).
17. D. M. Kessner, J. Singer, C. E. Kalk, and E. R. Schlesinger, *Contrasts in Health Status, vol. 1, Infant Death: An Analysis by Maternal Risk and Health Care* (Washington, D.C.: Institute of Medicine, National Academy of Sciences, 1973), pp. 96-122.
18. *Ibid.,* pp. 1-4.
19. U.S. Department of Health, Education and Welfare, National Center for Health Statistics, *Monthly Vital Statistics Report,* vol. 23, No. 11, DHEW Publication No. (HRA) 75-1120 (Washington, D.C.: U.S. Government Printing Office, 1975).
20. Shapiro, Schlesinger, and Nesbitt, *Infant, Perinatal, Maternal, and Childhood Mortality in the United States,* Table I-10A.
21. C. C. Dauer, R. F. Korns, and L. M. Schuman, *Infectious Diseases* (Cambridge, Mass.: Harvard University Press, 1968), pp. 60-63.
22. D. A. Boyes, The British Columbia screening program. *Obstetrical and Gynecological Survey* 24, 1005-11 (1969).
23. W. M. Christopherson, J. E. Parker, W. M. Mendez, and F. E. Lundin, Cervix cancer death rates and mass cytologic screening. *Cancer* 26, 808-11 (1970).
24. H. K. Fidler, D. A. Boyes, and A. J. Worth, Screening for malignant disease by exfoliative cytology, in *Presymptomatic Detection and Early Diagnosis: A Critical Appraisal,* eds. C. L. E. H. Sharp and H. Keen (Baltimore: Williams & Wilkins, 1968), pp. 295-336.
25. D. Schottenfeld, Patient risk factors and the detection of early cancer. *Preventive Medicine* 1, 335-51 (1972).
26. W. M. Christopherson and J. E. Parker, Control of cervix cancer in women of low income in a community. *Cancer* 24, 64-69 (1969).
27. F. E. Lundin, C. C. Erickson, and D. H. Sprunt, *Socioeconomic Dis-*

tribution of Cervical Cancer, in Relation to Early Marriage and Pregnancy, Public Health Monograph No. 73, P.H.S. Publication No. 1209 (Washington, D.C.: U.S. Government Printing Office, 1964).

28. T. Gordon and B. Devine, *Hypertension and Hypertensive Heart Disease in Adults, United States–1960–1962,* U.S. Department of Health, Education and Welfare, National Center for Health Statistics, P.H.S. Publication No. 1000, Series 11, No. 13 (Washington, D.C.: U.S. Government Printing Office, 1966).
29. Statistical Bulletin, Metropolitan Life, Reduced mortality from hypertension. *Statistical Bulletin* 53, 6-9 (May, 1972).
30. A. L. Cochrane, *Effectiveness and Efficiency: Random Reflections on Health Services* (Abingdon, England: The Nuffield Provincial Hospitals Trust, 1972), pp. 48-50.
31. A. G. Dingfelder, *Chronic Conditions Causing Activity Limitation, United States–July 1963–June 1965,* U.S. Department of Health, Education and Welfare, National Center for Health Statistics, P.H.S. Publication No. 1000, Series 10, No. 51 (Washington, D.C.: U.S. Government Printing Office, 1969).
32. A. B. Hollingshead and F. C. Redlich, *Social Class and Mental Illness: A Community Study* (New York: John Wiley & Sons, 1958), pp. 304-31.
33. E. L. White, *Personal Health Expenses, Per Capita Annual Expenses, United States–July–December, 1962,* U.S. Department of Health, Education and Welfare, National Center for Health Statistics, P.H.S. Publication No. 1000, Series 10, No. 27 (Washington, D.C.: U.S. Government Printing Office, 1966).
34. C. S. Wilder, *Family Use of Health Services, United States–July 1963–June 1964,* U.S. Department of Health, Education and Welfare, National Center for Health Statistics, P.H.S. Publication No. 1000, Series 10, No. 55 (Washington, D.C.: U.S. Government Printing Office, 1969).
35. A. J. Alderman, *Volume of Dental Visits, United States–July 1963–June 1964,* U.S. Department of Health, Education and Welfare, National Center for Health Statistics, P.H.S. Publication No. 1000, Series 10, No. 23 (Washington, D.C.: U.S. Government Printing Office, 1965).
36. M. S. Backenheimer, *Persons Hospitalized, by Number of Hospital Episodes and Days in a Year, United States–July 1965–June 1966,* U.S. Department of Health, Education and Welfare, National Center for Health Statistics, P.H.S. Publication, No. 1000, Series 10, No. 50 (Washington, D.C.: U.S. Government Printing Office, 1969).
37. J. K. Myers and L. L. Bean, *A Decade Later: A Follow-Up of Social Class and Mental Illness* (New York: John Wiley & Sons, 1968).
38. J. L. Dorsey, Physician distribution in Boston and Brookline: 1940 and 1961. *Medical Care* 7, 429-40 (1969).

39. R. Andersen and O. W. Anderson, *A Decade of Health Services: Social Survey Trends in Use and Expenditures* (Chicago: University of Chicago Press, 1967).
40. W. Winkelstein, Jr., and F. E. French, The role of ecology in the design of a health care system. *California Medicine* 113, 7-12 (1970).
41. L. Pratt, The relationship of socioeconomic status to health. *American Journal of Public Health* 61, 281-91 (1971).
42. N. B. Belloc, Relationship of health practices and mortality. *Preventive Medicine* 2, 67-81 (1973).
43. N. B. Belloc and L. Breslow, Relationship of physical health status and health practices. *Preventive Medicine* 1, 409-21 (1972).
44. D. Mechanic, *Public Expectations and Health Care* (New York: Wiley-Interscience, 1972).
45. E. Freidson, *Patients' Views of Medical Practice: A Study of Subscribers to a Prepaid Medical Plan in the Bronx* (New York: Russell Sage Foundation, 1961).
46. A. B. Ford, R. L. Liske, R. S. Ort, and J. C. Denton, *The Doctor's Perspective: Physicians View Their Patients and Practice* (Cleveland, Ohio: The Press of Case Western Reserve University, 1967), pp. 74-95.
47. R. Kohn, U.S. health facts: Toward an annual account of health and health services (Paper delivered at annual meeting of American Public Health Association, Atlantic City, New Jersey, November 13, 1972).
48. D. F. Sullivan, A single index of mortality and morbidity. *HSMHA Health Reports* 86, 347-54 (1971).
49. S. B. Goldsmith, The status of health status indicators. *Health Services Report* 87, 212-20 (1972).
50. N. B. Belloc, L. Breslow, and J. R. Hochstim, Measurement of physical health in a general population survey. *American Journal of Epidemiology* 93, 328-336 (1971).
51. P. A. Lembcke, Evolution of the medical audit. *Journal of the American Medical Association* 199, 543-50 (1967).
52. P. M. Densen, Public accountability and reporting systems in Medicare and other health programs. *New England Journal of Medicine* 289, 401-6 (1973).
53. B. A. Flashner, S. Reed, R. W. Coburn, and P. R. Fine, Professional standards review organizations: Analysis of their development and implementation based on a preliminary review of the hospital admission and surveillance program in Illinois. *Journal of the American Medical Association* 223, 1473-84 (1973).
54. M. Harrington, *Socialism* (New York: Saturday Review Press, 1972), p. 294.
55. H. B. Curry, Phoenix in flight: All systems go! *Journal of the American Medical Association* 222, 821-26 (1972).
56. R. M. Magraw, Trends in medical education and health services: Their

implications for a career in family medicine. *New England Journal of Medicine* 285, 1407-13 (1971).
57. A. M. Sadler, B. L. Sadler, and A. A. Bliss, *The Physician's Assistant, Today and Tomorrow* (New Haven: Yale University Press, 1972).

CHAPTER 7

1. U.S. Department of Commerce, Bureau of the Census, *Statistical Abstract of the United States, 1973,* 94th ed. (Washington, D.C.: U.S. Government Printing Office, 1973), Table 370; estimates of expenditure are based on distribution of population, health professionals, and hospitals presented in Chapter 5.
2. *Webster's Third New International Dictionary* (Springfield, Mass.: G. & C. Merriam Co., 1970).
3. E. Freidson, *Profession of Medicine* (New York: Dodd, Mead & Co., 1970).
4. D. K. Freeborn and B. J. Darsky, A study of the power structure of the medical community. *Medical Care* 12, 1-12 (1974).
5. J. G. Freymann, Leadership in American medicine: A matter of personal responsibility. *New England Journal of Medicine* 270, 710-20 (1964).
6. A. B. Ford, R. L. Liske, R. S. Ort, and J. C. Denton, *The Doctor's Perspective: Physicians View Their Patients and Practice* (Cleveland: The Press of Case Western Reserve University, 1967), pp. 143-47.
7. U.S. Department of Health, Education and Welfare, Public Health Service, *Health Manpower Source Book,* Section 20: Manpower supply and educational statistics for selected health occupations, P.H.S. Publication No. 263 (Washington, D.C.: U.S. Government Printing Office, 1969).
8. C. R. Rorem, *Private Group Clinics: The Administrative and Economic Aspects of Group Medical Practice,* Publication No. 8 (Washington, D.C.: The Committee on the Costs of Medical Care, 1931).
9. J. L. Schwartz, Early history of prepaid medical care plans. *Bulletin of the History of Medicine* 39, 450-75, 467-68 (1965).
10. L. T. Coggeshall, Planning for medical progress through education (a Report Submitted to the Executive Council of the Association of American Medical Colleges, A.A.M.C. 2530 Ridge Avenue, Evanston, Ill., April 1965).
11. American Medical Association, Council on Medical Education, Critique of the Coggeshall report—*Planning for Medical Progress through Education. Journal of the American Medical Association* 197, 909-12 (1966).
12. J. L. Dorsey, The prepaid group practice plan in the education of

future physicians: Initial efforts at the Harvard Community Health Plan. *Medical Care* 11, 12-20 (1973).
13. R. M. Heyssel, The Johns Hopkins-Columbia Medical Plan. *Medical Opinion and Review* 6, 30-37 (1970).
14. E. Ginzberg, and the Conservation of Human Resources Staff, Columbia University, *Urban Health Services: The Case of New York* (New York: Columbia University Press, 1971), pp. 96-118.
15. M. Cherkasky, The hospital as a social instrument: Recent experiences at Montefiore Hospital, in *Hospitals, Doctors, and the Public Interest,* ed. J. H. Knowles (Cambridge, Mass.: Harvard University Press, 1965), pp. 93-110.
16. R. Stevens, *American Medicine and the Public Interest* (New Haven, Conn.: Yale University Press, 1971).
17. R. H. Ebert, The role of the medical school in planning the health-care system. *Journal of Medical Education* 42, 481-88 (1967).
18. U.S. Department of Health, Education and Welfare, Public Health Service, *Health Manpower Source Book,* Section 21: Allied Health Manpower, 1950-80, P.H.S. Publication No. 263, Sec. 21 (Washington, D.C.: U.S. Government Printing Office, 1970).
19. A. M. Sadler, B. L. Sadler, and A. A. Bliss, *The Physician's Assistant: Today and Tomorrow* (New Haven, Conn.: Yale University Press, 1972).
20. A. B. Ford and D. F. Ransohoff, *The Contribution of Non-physician Health Workers to the Delivery of Primary Care* (Department of Community Health, Case Western Reserve University School of Medicine, Cleveland, Ohio, 1971).
21. E. Ginzberg, *Men, Money, and Medicine* (New York: Columbia University Press, 1969), pp. 60-72.
22. R. S. Duff and A. B. Hollingshead, *Sickness and Society* (New York: Harper & Row, 1968).
23. J. O. Hepner and D. M. Hepner, *The Health Strategy Game: A Challenge for Reorganization and Management* (St. Louis: C. V. Mosby, 1973).
24. B. S. Cooper, N. L. Worthington, and P. A. Piro, National health expenditures, 1929-73. *Social Security Bulletin* 37, 3-49 (1974).
25. U.S. Department of Health, Education and Welfare, Public Health Service, *Health Manpower Source Book,* Section 20: Manpower Supply and Educational Statistics for Selected Health Occupations, P.H.S. Publication No. 263 (Washington, D.C.: U.S. Government Printing Office, 1969), Table 33.
26. D. L. Rabin, B. H. Starfield, C. F. Burns, J. R. Krasno, and M. C. McCormick, Estimated physician services in a United States metropolitan area. *International Journal of Health Services* 3, 197-211 (1973).
27. B. Ehrenreich and J. Ehrenreich, *The American Health Empire:*

Power, Profits and Politics (New York: Random House, 1971), pp. 50-61.

28. Darling v. Charleston Memorial Hospital, 33 Illinois 2nd 326 N.E. 2nd 253 (1965); certiorari denied 383 U.S. 946 (1966).
29. Hepner and Hepner, *The Health Strategy Game: A Challenge for Reorganization and Management,* pp. 289-294.
30. J. H. Knowles, The balanced biology of the teaching hospital, in *Hospitals, Doctors, and the Public Interest,* ed. J. H. Knowles (Cambridge, Mass.: Harvard University Press, 1965), pp. 34-37.
31. J. K. Galbraith, *The New Industrial State* (New York: The New American Library, 1967), p. 69.
32. R. H. Egdahl, Foundations for medical care. *New England Journal of Medicine* 288, 491-98 (1973).
33. National Commission on Community Health Services, *Health is a Community Affair* (Cambridge, Mass.: Harvard University Press, 1966), pp. 151-66.
34. Ray H. Elling and Ollie J. Lee, Formal connections of community leadership to the health system. *Milbank Memorial Foundation Quarterly* 44, 294-306 (1966).
35. W. D. Callender, Jr., The impact of federal legislation on voluntary agencies. *Community* (November–December, 1969), pp. 3-6.
36. W. S. Clark, The voluntary health movement in transition. *Rehabilitation Literature* 31, 135-39 (1970).
37. S. E. Harris, Economics of drugs, in *The Economics of American Medicine* (New York: Macmillan, 1964), pp. 73-103.
38. H. M. Somers and A. R. Somers, The new role of the drug industry, in *Doctors, Patients, and Health Insurance: The Organization and Financing of Medical Care* (Garden City, New York: Doubleday, 1961), pp. 81-92.
39. Ehrenreich and Ehrenreich, *The American Health Empire: Power, Profits, and Politics,* pp. 95-123.
40. Cooper, Worthington, and Piro, National health expenditures, 1929–73. *Social Security Bulletin.*
41. H. M. Somers and A. R. Somers, *Medicare and the Hospitals: Issues and Prospects* (Washington, D.C.: The Brookings Institution, 1967), p. 63.
42. S. A. Law, *Blue Cross: What Went Wrong?* (New Haven, Conn.: Yale University Press, 1974).
43. Somers and Somers, *Medicare and the Hospitals: Issues and Prospects,* pp. 155-58.
44. Ehrenreich and Ehrenreich, *The American Health Empire: Power, Profits, and Politics,* pp. 147-63.
45. Somers and Somers, *Medicare and the Hospitals: Issues and Prospects,* p. 23.
46. Ginzberg, *Urban Health Services: The Case of New York,* pp. 206-24.

47. Cooper, Worthington, and Piro, National health expenditures, 1929-73.
48. U.S. Department of Health, Education and Welfare, Public Health Service, National Center for Health Statistics, *Health Resources Statistics, 1972-73* (Washington, D.C.: U.S. Government Printing Office, 1973), pp. 23-26.
49. Somers and Somers, *Doctors, Patients, and Health Insurance: The Organization and Financing of Medical Care,* pp. 496-505.
50. J. L. Schwartz, Early history of prepaid medical care plans. *Bulletin of the History of Medicine* 39, 451-52 (1965).
51. Somers and Somers, *Doctors, Patients, and Health Insurance: The Organization and Financing of Medical Care,* pp. 207-14.
52. *Ibid.,* pp. 308-9, 323-25.
53. Ginzberg, *Urban Health Services: The Case of New York,* p. 144.
54. Teamster Center Program, *A Study of the Quality of Hospital Care Secured by A Sample of Teamster Family Members in New York City* (New York: Columbia University School of Public Health and Administrative Medicine, 1964).
55. Hepner and Hepner, *The Health Strategy Game: A Challenge for Reorganization and Management,* pp. 74-79.
56. D. P. Moynihan, *Maximum Feasible Misunderstanding: Community Action in the War on Poverty* (New York: The Free Press, 1969).
57. A. B. Shostak, The future of poverty, *Poverty and Health: A Sociological Analysis,* eds. J. Kosa, A. Antonovsky, and I. K. Zola (Cambridge, Mass.: Harvard University Press, 1969), pp. 274-79.
58. Hepner and Hepner, *The Health Strategy Game: A Challenge for Reorganization and Management,* pp. 37-39.
59. H. Notkin and M. S. Notkin, Community participation in health services: A review article. *Medical Care Review* 27, 1178-1201 (1970).
60. R. Fein, The new national health spending policy. *New England Journal of Medicine* 290, 137-40 (1974).
61. Ginzberg, *Urban Health Services: The Case of New York,* p. 224.
62. Galbraith, *The New Industrial State,* p. 67.
63. Hepner and Hepner, *The Health Strategy Game: A Challenge for Reorganization and Management,* pp. 286-89.
64. A. R. Somers, *Health Care in Transition: Directions for the Future* (Chicago, Ill.: Hospital Research and Educational Trust, 1971).
65. D. D. Rutstein, *Blueprint for Medical Care* (Cambridge, Mass.: MIT Press, 1974).
66. C. D. Gibson, Jr., Will the urban university medical center join the community? *Journal of Medical Education* 45, 144-48 (1970).

CHAPTER 8

1. R. Harris, *A Sacred Trust* (New York: New American Library, 1966).
2. K. L. White, J. H. Murnaghan, and C. R. Gaus, Technology and health care. *New England Journal of Medicine* 287, 1223-27 (1972).
3. R. M. Battistella and T. E. Chester, Role of management in health services in Britain and the United States. *Lancet* 1, 626-30 (1972).
4. E. A. Krause, Health planning as a managerial ideology. *International Journal of Health Services* 3, 445-63 (1973).
5. M. I. Roemer and J. W. Friedman, *Doctors in Hospitals: Medical Staff Organization and Hospital Performance* (Baltimore: The Johns Hopkins Press, 1971).
6. B. A. Flashner, S. Reed, R. W. Coburn, and P. R. Fine, Professional standards review organizations. *Journal of the American Medical Association* 223, 1473-84 (1973).
7. E. D. Acheson, *Record Linkage in Medicine: Proceedings of the International Symposium, Oxford, July 1967* (London: E. & S. Livingstone Ltd., 1968).
8. L. L. Weed, *Medical Records, Medical Education, and Patient Care: The Problem-Oriented Record as a Basic Tool* (Cleveland: Press of Case Western Reserve University, 1969).
9. J. O. Hepner and D. M. Hepner, *The Health Strategy Game: A Challenge for Reorganization and Management* (St. Louis: C. J. Mosby, 1973), pp. 252-58.
10. A. de Tocqueville, *Democracy in America,* trans. G. Lawrence; ed. J. P. Mayer (Garden City, New York: Doubleday, 1969), p. 693.
11. National Commission on Community Health Services, *Health is a Community Affair* (Cambridge, Mass.: Harvard University Press, 1966).
12. U.S. Public Health Service, Health Services and Mental Health Administration, Community Health Service, *The Urban Planner in Health Planning: A Report by the American Society of Planning Officials,* P.H.S. Publication No. 1888 (Washington, D.C.: U.S. Government Printing Office, 1968).
13. U.S. Department of Health, Education and Welfare, Human Investments Program, *Delivery of Health Services for the Poor* (Washington, D.C.: U.S. Government Printing Office, 1967).
14. T. E. Bryant, Goals and potential of the neighborhood health centers (editorial). *Medical Care* 8, 93-94 (1970).
15. J. D. Stoeckle and L. M. Candib, The neighborhood health center—Reform ideas of yesterday and today. *New England Journal of Medicine* 280, 1385-91 (1969).
16. E. Feingold, A political scientist's view of the neighborhood health center as a new social institution. *Medical Care* 8, 108-15 (1970).
17. L. W. Cronkhite, Jr., What are the conflicts involved in community

control? in *Medicine in the Ghetto,* ed. John C. Norman (New York: Appleton-Century-Crofts, 1969), pp. 283-89.
18. M. A. Morehead, Evaluating quality of medical care in the neighborhood health center program of the Office of Economic Opportunity. *Medical Care* 8, 118-31 (1970).
19. M. A. Morehead, R. S. Donaldson, and M. R. Seravalli, Comparisons between OEO neighborhood health centers and other health care providers of ratings of the quality of health care. *American Journal of Public Health* 61, 1294-1306 (1971).
20. R. J. Blendon and C. R. Gaus, Problems in developing health services in poverty areas: The Johns Hopkins experience. *Journal of Medical Education* 46, 477-84 (1971).
21. D. L. Cowen, Denver's neighborhood health program. *Public Health Reports* 84, 1027-31 (1969).
22. R. Fein, An economist's view of the neighborhood health center as a new social institution. *Medical Care* 8, 104-7 (1971).
23. R. D. Fraser, An international study of health and general systems of financing health care, *International Journal of Health Services* 3, 369-97 (1973).
24. *New York Times,* City's year-old abortion record hailed (June 30, 1971), p. 37.
25. J. Jacobs, *The Economy of Cities* (New York: Vintage Books, 1970).
26. E. Howard, *Garden Cities of Tomorrow* (originally published 1898), ed. F. J. Osborn (London: Faber and Faber, 1965).
27. R. M. Heyssel, The Johns Hopkins–Columbia Medical Plan. *Medical Opinion and Review* (January, 1970), pp. 30-37.
28. W. S. Fiser, The lesson of Toronto, in *Metropolis: Values in Conflict,* eds. C. E. Elias, Jr., J. Gillies, and S. Riemer (Belmont, Calif.: Wadsworth Publishing Co., 1964), pp. 277-80.

CHAPTER 9

1. J. H. de Haas and J. H. de Haas-Posthuma, Sociomedical achievements in the People's Republic of China. *International Journal of Health Services* 3, 275-94 (1973).
2. V. W. Sidel and R. Sidel, *Serve the People: Observations on Medicine in the People's Republic of China* (New York: Josiah Macy, Jr., Foundation, 1973).
3. M. Stanley, Two experiences of an American public health nurse in China a quarter of a century apart. *American Journal of Public Health* 63, 111-16 (1973).
4. M. E. Wegman, T. Lin, and E. F. Purcell (eds.), *Public Health in the People's Republic of China* (New York: Josiah Macy, Jr., Foundation, 1973).

5. H. Ågren, Medical practice in China: A compendium (book review). *Science* 178, 394-95 (1972).
6. L. Huberman and P. M. Sweezy, *Socialism in Cuba* (New York: Monthly Review Press, 1969), pp. 53-64.
7. V. Navarro, Health services in Cuba: An initial appraisal. *New England Journal of Medicine* 287, 954-59 (1972).
8. Milton I. Roemer, Political ideology and health care: Hospital practice in the Phillipines and Cuba. *International Journal of Health Services* 3, 487-92 (1973).
9. Wegman, Lin, and Purcell, eds., *Public Health in the People's Republic of China,* p. 261.
10. R. J. Bazell, Health radicals: Crusade to shift medical power to the people, *Science* 173, 506-9 (1971).
11. B. Ehrenreich and J. Ehrenreich, *The American Health Empire: Power, Profits, and Politics* (New York: Random House, 1971), pp. 27-28.
12. H. Waitzkin and B. Waterman, *The Exploitation of Illness in Capitalist Society* (Indianapolis: Bobbs-Merrill, 1974).
13. I. Illich, *Medical Nemesis: The Expropriation of Health* (London, Calder and Boyars, 1975).
14. These ideas are drawn from several sources, particularly *Health Rights News,* Editorial, May/June, 1971 and Waitzkin and Waterman, *The Exploitation of Illness in Capitalist Society,* pp. 108-16.
15. S. Wolfe, Health and the 1972 U.S. election: Postmortem with rigor mortis. *International Journal of Health Services* 3, 319-326 (1973).
16. D. E. Smith, Runaways and their health problems in Haight-Ashbury during the summer of 1967. *American Journal of Public Health* 59, 2046-50 (1969).
17. J. D. Stoeckle, W. H. Anderson, J. Page, and J. Brenner, The free medical clinics. *Journal of the American Medical Association* 219, 603-5 (1972).
18. W. C. McWilliams, *The Idea of Fraternity in America* (Berkeley: University of California Press, 1973).
19. M. I. Roemer and W. Shonick, HMO performance: The recent evidence, health and society. *Milbank Memorial Fund Quarterly* 51, 271-317 (1973).
20. A. Donabedian, An evaluation of prepaid group practice. *Inquiry* 6, 3-27 (1969).
21. C. R. Rorem, *Private Group Clinics,* The Committee on the Costs of Medical Care, Publication No. 8 (Chicago: University of Chicago Press, 1931), pp. 95ff (reprinted by Milbank Memorial Fund, 1971).
22. E. W. Saward, *The Relevance of Prepaid Group Practice to the Effective Delivery of Health Services,* U.S. Department of Health, Education and Welfare, Public Health Service (Washington, D.C.: U.S. Government Printing Office, 1970).

23. R. L. Bashshur, C. A. Metzner, and C. Worden, Consumer satisfaction with group practice, the CHA case. *American Journal of Public Health* 57, 1991-99 (1967).
24. S. Wolfe and R. F. Badgley, *The Family Doctor* (New York: Milbank Memorial Fund, 1972), pp. 102, 113.
25. M. E. McNamara and C. Todd, A survey of group practice in the United States, 1969. *American Journal of Public Health* 60, 1303-13 (1970).
26. Wolfe and Badgley, *The Family Doctor,* pp. 117-118.
27. Donabedian, An evaluation of prepaid group practice, pp. 3-27.
28. Special Task Force, *Work in America: Report of a Special Task Force to the Secretary of Health, Education and Welfare* (Cambridge, Mass.: MIT Press, 1973), pp. 93-120.
29. H. Wise, R. Beckhard, I. Rubin, and A. L. Kyte, *Making Health Teams Work* (Cambridge, Mass.: Ballinger Publishing Co., 1974).
30. A. S. Golden, D. G. Carlson, and B. Harris, Jr., Non-physician family health teams for health maintenance organizations. *American Journal of Public Health* 63, 732-36 (1973).
31. R. Beckhard, Organizational issues in the team delivery of comprehensive health care, Part 1. *Milbank Memorial Fund Quarterly* 50 (3), 287-316 (1972).
32. I. M. Rubin and R. Beckhard, Factors influencing the effectiveness of health teams, Part 1. *Milbank Memorial Fund Quarterly* 50 (3), 317-35 (1972).
33. B. Bates, Physician and nurse practitioner: Conflict and reward. *Annals of Internal Medicine* 82, 702-6 (1975).
34. P. M. Newton and D. J. Levinson, The work group within the organization: A sociopsychological approach. *Psychiatry* 36, 115-42 (1973).
35. American Medical Association, *Directory of Approved Internships and Residencies, 1973–74* (Chicago: American Medical Association, 1973), pp. 370-72.
36. L. H. Andrus and J. P. Geyman, Managing the health care team, in *Family Practice,* eds. H. F. Conn, R. E. Rakel, and T. W. Johnson (Philadelphia: W. B. Saunders Co., 1973), pp. 139-58.
37. J. P. Geyman, *The Modern Family Doctor and Changing Medical Practice* (New York: Appleton-Century-Crofts, 1971), pp. 174-88.
38. G. A. Silver, *Family Medical Care: A Design for Health Maintenance* (Cambridge, Mass.: Ballinger Publishing Co., 1974).
39. E. Freidson, *Patients' Views of Medical Practice* (New York: Russell Sage Foundation, 1961).
40. S. W. Bloom, *The Doctor and His Patient: A Sociological Interpretation* (New York: Free Press, 1965).
41. H. E. Vandervoort and D. C. Ransom, Undergraduate education in family medicine. *Journal of Medical Education* 48, 158-65 (1973).

42. J. I. Williams and T. L. Leaman, Family structure and function, in *Family Practice,* eds. H. F. Conn, R. E. Rakel, and T. W. Johnson (Philadelphia: W. B. Saunders Co., 1973), pp. 3-18.
43. E. F. Schumacher, *Small is Beautiful: A Study of Economics as if People Mattered* (New York: Harper & Row, 1973).
44. *Ibid.,* pp. 70, 62, and 31-32.
45. McWilliams, *The Idea of Fraternity in America,* pp. 7-8.
46. H. F. Harlow and M. K. Harlow, The affectional systems, in *Behavior of Nonhuman Primates,* eds. A. M. Schrier, H. F. Harlow, and F. Stollnitz (New York: Academic Press, 1965), Vol. 2, pp. 287-334.

APPENDIX A

1. L. Wirth, Urbanism as a way of life. *American Journal of Sociology* 44, 1-24 (1938). Reprinted in *American Urban History,* ed. A. B. Callow, Jr. (New York: Oxford University Press, 1969), pp. 488-503.
2. H. J. Gans, Urbanism and suburbanism as ways of life: A re-evaluation of definitions, in *Human Behavior and Social Processes,* ed. Arnold Rose (Boston: Houghton Mifflin, 1962), pp. 625-48.
3. A. Toynbee, *Cities on the Move* (New York: Oxford University Press, 1970), p. 13.
4. L. Mumford, *The City in History* (Harmondsworth, Middlesex, England: Penguin Books, 1961), p. 11.
5. S. Milgram, The experience of living in cities. *Science* 167, 1461-68 (1970).
6. K. Davis, The urbanization of the human population, *Cities: A 'Scientific American' Book* (Harmondsworth, Middlesex, England: Penguin Books, 1967), pp. 11-32.
7. H. Blumenfeld, The modern metropolis, in *Cities: A 'Scientific American' Book* (Harmondsworth, Middlesex, England: Penguin Books, 1967), pp. 49-66.
8. J. Jacobs, The kind of problem a city is, in *The Death and Life of Great American Cities* (New York: Random House, 1961), pp. 428-48.
9. C. A. Doxiadis, *Ekistics: An Introduction to the Science of Human Settlements* (New York, Oxford University Press, 1968).
10. R. L. Meier, The metropolis as a transaction-maximizing system. *Daedalus* (Fall, 1968) (The Conscience of the City), pp. 1292-1313.
11. D. L. Birch, *The Economic Future of City and Suburb,* Committee for Economic Development, Supplementary Paper No. 30 (New York: Committee for Economic Development, 1970).
12. U.S. Department of Commerce, National Bureau of Standards, Fed-

eral Information Processing Standards Publication No. 8-4, Standard Metropolitan Statistical Areas (Washington, D.C.: U.S. Government Printing Office, 1974).

13. U.S. Department of Commerce, Bureau of the Census, Current Population Reports, *Consumer Income,* Series P-60, No. 66, December 23, 1969.
14. J. Storck, *Report of the Twentieth Anniversary Conference of the United States National Committee on Vital and Health Statistics,* U.S. Department of Health, Education and Welfare, National Center for Health Statistics, P.H.S. Publication No. 1000, Series 4, No. 13 (Washington, D.C.: U.S. Government Printing Office, 1970).
15. N. E. Manos, *Comparative Mortality among Metropolitan Areas of the United States, 1949–51,* Public Health Service, Bureau of State Services, Division of Special Health Services, Air Pollution Medical Program, P.H.S. Publication No. 562 (Washington, D.C.: U.S. Government Printing Office, 1957).
16. E. A. Duffy and R. E. Carroll, *United States Metropolitan Mortality, 1959–1961,* P.H.S. Publication No. 999-AP-39, U.S. Public Health Service, National Center for Air Pollution Control, 1957.
17. E. M. Kitagawa and P. M. Hauser, *Differential Mortality in the United States: A Study in Socioeconomic Epidemiology* (Cambridge, Mass.: Harvard University Press, 1973).
18. These data have been furnished for this study by The National Center for Health Statistics.
19. R. D. Grove and A. M. Hetzel, *Vital Statistics Rates in the United States 1940–1960,* U.S. Department of Health, Education and Welfare, Public Health Service, National Center for Health Statistics (Washington, D.C.: U.S. Government Printing Office, 1968).
20. P. W. Haberman, The reliability of the data, in *Poverty and Health,* eds. J. Kosa, A. Antonovsky, and I. K. Zola (Cambridge, Mass.: Harvard University Press, 1969), pp. 343-83.
21. S. Shapiro and J. Unger, *Weight at Birth and Survival of the Newborn, by Geographic Divisions and Urban and Rural Areas, United States, Early 1950,* U.S. Department of Health, Education and Welfare, National Center for Health Statistics, P.H.S. Publication No. 1000, Series 21, No. 4 (Washington, D.C.: U.S. Government Printing Office, 1965).
22. E. W. Curran, *Report of the International Conference on the Perinatal and Infant Mortality Problem of the United States,* U.S. Department of Health, Education and Welfare, National Center for Health Statistics, P.H.S. Publication No. 1000, Series 4, No. 3 (Washington, D.C.: U.S. Government Printing Office, 1966).
23. K. E. Taeuber, L. Chiazze, Jr., and W. Haenzel, *Migration in the United States: An Analysis of Residence Histories,* Public Health Monograph No. 77, P.H.S. Publication No. 1575 (Washington, D.C.: U.S. Government Printing Office, 1968).

24. U.S. Department of Commerce, Bureau of the Census, Current Population Reports, Series P-20, Washington, D.C.
25. C. W. Namey and R. W. Wilson, *Health Characteristics by Geographic Region, Large Metropolitan Areas, and Other Places of Residence, United States–1969–70,* U.S. Department of Health, Education and Welfare, National Center for Health Statistics, Vital and Health Statistics, Series 10, No. 86, DHEW Publication No. (HRA) 74-1513 (Washington, D.C.: U.S. Government Printing Office, 1974).
26. Henry W. Miller, *Plan and Operation of the Health and Nutrition Examination Survey, United States–1971–1973,* U.S. Department of Health, Education and Welfare, National Center for Health Statistics, Vital and Health Statistics, Series 1, No. 10a, DHEW Publication No. (HSM) 73-1310 (Washington, D.C.: U.S. Government Printing Office, 1973).
27. F. E. Linder, The health of the American people. *Scientific American* 214 (6), 21-29 (1966).
28. U.S. Department of Health, Education and Welfare, National Center for Health Statistics, Vital and Health Statistics, Series 2: Data Evaluation and Methods Research.

INDEX

Page numbers for figures and tables are in **boldface** type